CANCER SOLUTIONS: RIFE, ENERGY MEDICINE, AND MEDICAL POLITICS

Written by Barry Lynes

Author of

The Cancer Cure That Worked: The Rife Report

First printing March 1987
Second printing January 1989
Third printing August 1989
Fourth printing April 1992
Fifth printing August 1994
Sixth printing October 1997
Seventh printing June 1999
Eighth printing August 2000

ISBN: 1-8852730-9-6

Published by:
Elsmere Press
P.O. Box 130
Delmar, NY 12054
www.ElsmerePress.com

"Never doubt that a small group of thoughtful committed citizens can change the world; indeed it's the only thing that ever does."
Margaret Mead, noted anthropologist

"Here is the key to our policy — the right to choose. Human beings everywhere simply as an inalienable right of birth, should have freedom to choose their guiding philosophy, their form of government, their methods of progress. The right of the individual to elect freely the manner of his care in illness must be preserved."
Dwight David Eisenhower, President of the United States of America 1953-1961

"It is from numberless diverse acts of courage and belief that human history is shaped. Each time a man stands up for an ideal, or acts to improve the lot of others, or strikes out against injustice, he sends a tiny ripple of hope, and crossing each other from a million different centers of energy and daring, these ripples build a current which can sweep down the mightiest walls of oppression and resistance."
Robert F. Kennedy, Attorney General of the United States of America; also United States Senator representing the state of New York

"We have always been very interested in the future... a very American trait... Because the future was going to be better... And that's the kick. It's the discovery. It's the adventure that comes

with discovery and getting on a project and finding things out yourself. It's suddenly seeing things come into focus and realizing, 'Oh, my goodness, look at this. Yes, I see. I understand now.'"

David McCullouch, noted historian

"The medicine of the future will be energy medicine. Probably 80 percent of medicine will be energy medicine, and 20 percent chemical medicine."

Dr. Robert Jacobs, Natural Products Pharmacologist

"To me, the future of medicine is in light and electromagnetic fields... once we find a way of manipulating and controlling electromagnetic fields, we will be able to cure just about any disease... Probably the guy who knew the most was Royal Raymond Rife."

Dr. Francisco Contreras, Oncology Surgeon, Oasis Hospital

"This is how tyrannies end: when people stop fearing the tyrant."

Jean-Louis Gassee, President & Founder of Be, Inc.

Table Of Contents

Author's Preface

This is a very serious book. There are charges and there are documented facts in here that responsible readers will not simply read, shrug, say "that's interesting," or deny because they don't like what has been put before their eyes and now is a part of their awareness. The key word is responsible. Of course, a vast majority will do any or all of the other options. I do not write for this vast majority. I write for those who do take this kind of unnecessary mass suffering and death as something not to be excused, ignored, denied or, at minimum, discarded with some superficial excuse or argument.

There is evidence — factual and documented — which clearly, carefully cries out for attention and deep regard from serious, responsible men and women who hold important public and private sector positions.

You, the reader of this book, are about to go on a journey. It will not be a pleasant trip. You do not have to go. You do not have to read this book. But, if you do read this book, be mindful that you are dealing with very real dilemmas, very real corruption, terrible wrongs from a system dangerous to the health of the American public and indeed, the entire global community — of which the American nation is both a part and a leader.

Evil actions, evil men and women, tyrannical professional groups, and self-serving commercial interests which extract murderous costs in order to profit cannot be ignored or permitted to continue their exploitive ways forever. There always come days of accounting, judgment, justice and fundamental reckoning followed by permanent change in how things are done — how medicine will be done in the future, how science will be conducted in the future, how government health officials will put the public interest first, or else they will have to answer for both deeds and omissions. All this is coming as surely as the sun will rise explained in this book will be ended. That is guaranteed. Sooner or later, with or without each of you who read this book and learn from it, the evil will be ended.

Your journey begins on the next page.

Quotes in this book have been edited for clarity.

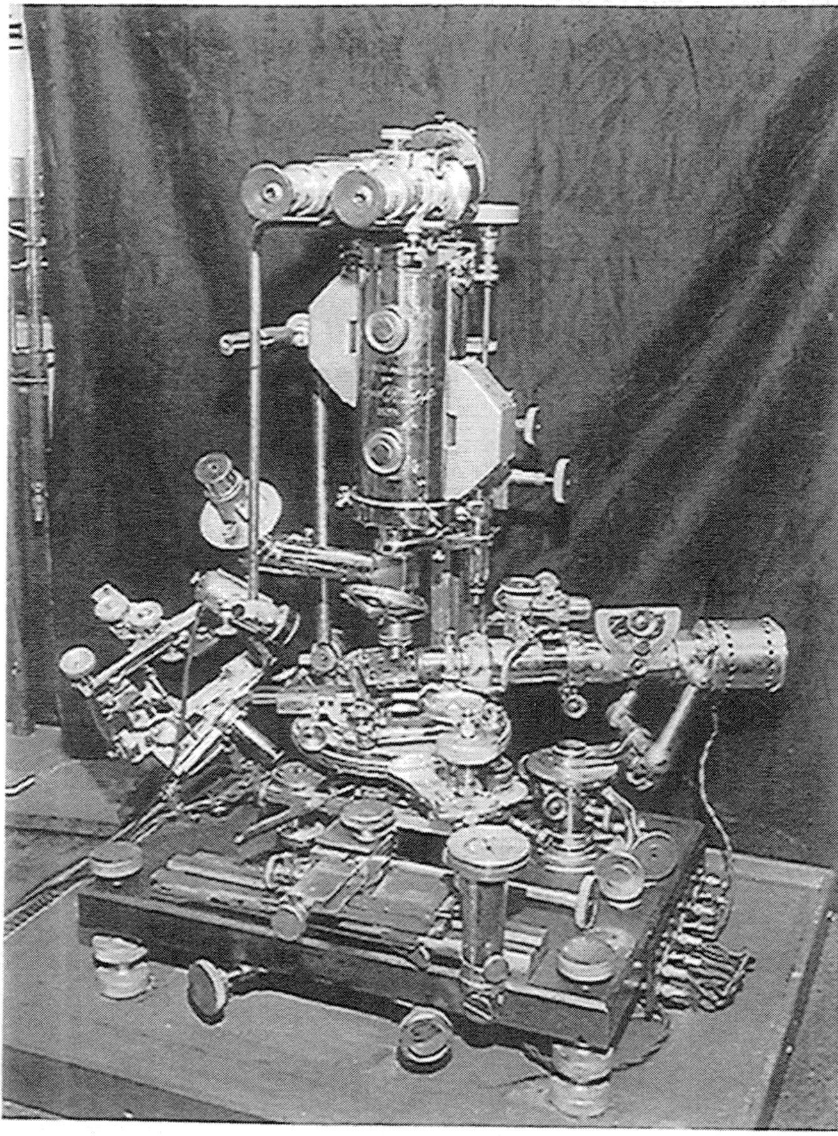

Royal Rife's Light Microscope

Foreword

A number of cures for cancer and other diseases have been ignored or suppressed by medical interests. This has occurred throughout the 20th century and has been particularly virulent and abusive of patients, unconventional scientists, and alternative physicians during the decade of the 1990's.

Historians of the future undoubtedly will describe in great detail how the medical and scientific elite of America, as well as their counterparts in other countries, conspired to maintain a monopoly despite terrible, genocidal level torture and death for so many innocent victims who trusted their doctors.

Even as the alternative health movement grew enormously in the 1990's and the documentation proving decades of medical malevolence became available to more citizens via the various communication revolutions, those directing and monopolizing mainstream medicine denounced and fought furiously against what the hard evidence clearly proved. The reality of a medical-scientific-government health bureaucracy network in collusion and actively suppressing breakthrough healing science, healing arts, and inexpensive, simple-to-use therapies was an established fact. Those with medical monopoly powers refused to honor basic scientific principles, the Hippocratic Oath, and obligations of government officials to be accountable.

This foul betrayal of people's basic rights to have honest health information and access to quality alternative therapies constitutes a crime of monumental, historic proportions and a political evil that must be corrected if civilization is to move forward.

The critical mass building to an explosive showdown resembles other great turning points of Western Civilization such as the establishment of citizen rights, the end of slavery, the overthrow of religious absolutism, the women's right to vote, the birth of scientific rules, and open, public debate on great issues or national policies.

If you, the reader, care about your health and the future progress of civilization, this book has both a personal and a societal message for you. It is a simple and a hard message: Be aware that your lives and the lives of your loved ones are now threatened by an invisible, medical tyranny as dangerous and evil as those brought by Hitler and Stalin in other times.

A furious battle has been raging for decades and continues to be fought in the arena of orthodox versus alternative health practices. Most of these battles have occurred behind-the-scenes as a small group of science "insiders," highly political doctor groups, high government health officials, and commercial interests in the private sector have actively conspired to keep a corrupt, tyrannical system in place. They have protected their own financially lucrative careers at the public's expense. They sneer at, denounce, and, using powerful public relations organizations, attack a variety of new scientific tools and healing therapies. It is a self-serving, evil agenda they pursue. It is possible — naively — to claim they are merely ignorant of new realities. The documented facts, gathered over many years, clearly show conscious efforts by self-serving medical and scientific interests to destroy or suppress valid scientific and healing discoveries which might disrupt or replace the existing orthodoxies.

When the forces of progressive civilization win — as they will win — the next phase of human evolution will commence. Until that revolution has happened, a terrible toll in human suffering and human lives will continue.

When this scandal of medical science finally erupts into the mass consciousness and all the games, all the politics, and at least some of the dirty deeds of the government health bureaucrats, the medical associations and other "interested" parties are revealed, it is likely that a revulsion and fury will burst forth from the general American public and decent people around the world.

CHAPTER 1: ROYAL R. RIFE

In the spring of 1987 a small paperback book of 167 pages, which I authored, quietly, unobtrusively entered the world through a small publishing company in Canada. *The Cancer Cure That Worked: The Rife Report* told the story of Royal R. Rife, a San Diego, California scientist whose laboratory, discoveries, and inventions stirred excited talk between many prominent scientists and doctors in the 1930's.

Rife had invented a super light microscope which enabled him to view live, virus-size microbes. This invention shattered all the acknowledged laws and principles of microscopy and physics.

Today, as the 20th century ends and the 21st century is born, orthodox scientists and microscope experts cannot equal Rife's accomplishment of 70 years earlier!

The electron microscope obtains great magnification and resolution, but the electrons bombarding the tiny, disease-causing microbes kill them, and standard light microscopes must use killing chemical stains. The problem of observing dead microbes remains. Plus, standard light microscopes, governed by rigidly limiting laws of physics, obtain extremely low magnification and resolution. Thus the significance of Rife's invention was monumental. Rife's uniquely designed light microscope soared into unbelievable regions of magnification and resolution.

Rife's light microscope enabled him and the other scientists and doctors who were at his side to see live microbes of virus size! This enabled them to use various, specific electronic frequencies to destroy or devitalize safely and painlessly the cause of many human diseases. A revolutionary approach to healing was thus born in Royal R. Rife's San Diego, California laboratory during the 1930s.

His inventions could have altered the direction of all of 20th century
science!

Unfortunately, there were medical and scientific interests who did not want Rife's great discovery to become public knowledge and develop into mainstream medical procedures and therapies. It was too simple and too inexpensive. Medical interests and powerful scientific orthodoxies were threatened. Payoffs, combined with active opposition and censorship, resulted in the suppression of Rife and his work. A great wall descended around Rife and all his historic accomplishments. He became "invisible" just as many political figures in the old Soviet Union did during its tyranny — except, this was in the United States of America!

Royal R. Rife died in 1971, a forgotten and broken man.

Yet, he had bequeathed a great legacy, possibly as wonderful and lasting as those given to humanity by Galileo, Martin Luther and other giants who were attacked in their time, but later were recognized as geniuses and heroes of a very rare, special kind. Rife's work and Rife's discoveries did not die with him. Rife now "*speaks to the centuries.*" The revolution he helped to birth in the 1930's thrives as the 20th century concludes and the 21st century opens.

Many people who suffer from cancer, herpes, tuberculosis and other diseases are now being cured using Rife therapies. Much of the therapy occurs underground at the grassroots level. Some people are exploiting the Rife legacy and offering dubious devices which accomplish nothing for desperate, sick people. Conversely, a number of dedicated engineers, scientists, physicians and alternative health practitioners are offering quality Rife instruments, Rife-inspired (but different) devices and approaches, or basic Rife procedures integrated into a larger complementary program to restore patient health or at least restrain disease degeneration.

Still others have gone far beyond Rife. Unbelievable results are being obtained quietly in a few locations despite active, organized suppression by commercial interests and orthodox scientific, medical and governmental forces.

In other words, a great struggle and revolution has been underway since 1987 when the Rife book was first published. A virulent effort by orthodox medical and scientific forces, aided by government bureaucrats and mysterious private interests, continues to suppress what could clearly benefit millions and millions of people throughout the world.

CHAPTER 2: WHY A REVOLUTION NOW?

This is a book about American politics and dirty deeds in the insulated sphere of American medicine and medical science. Yet, people in many nations can benefit by knowing the awful truths told here. This book is about suppression of cures for diseases as well as cures for various addictions (including drugs). The suppressions occurred so that a few powerful interests could continue to profit from the existing status quo. This book is about corruption and evil in high places. This book is about a fearful, timid media watching out for its own interests rather than serving the public interest. That means this book accuses highly paid editors and journalists of avoiding the tough stories even though millions of lives could be saved and terrible suffering avoided if those directly controlling the international, national and local media dared to break the wall of silence concerning medical crimes.

This is a book which asks that a minimal concern for the public interest be recognized in these cynical, commercial times. The public interest is perceived and defined here as real, flesh and blood human beings undergoing indescribable agonies. Why is this happening? Because the few who have the obligation to report the truth about conscious, organized medical mischief choose instead to protect their media careers, play safe corporate politics, and serve as public relations flunkies for the medical interests.

Mostly, this book is about medical science gone bad — dishonest, political, and filled with disinformation — pouring its errors, its corrupt bargains, and its monumental ignorance onto an unsuspecting public and deeply into the brains of students who will become tomorrow's doctors and scientists.

Thus, as the 20th century closes and a new century dawns, a revolution born of revulsion against evil medical and scientific patterns of behavior grows. This active, grassroots movement challenges the existing orthodox medical-scientific world as totally as Galileo broke the cozy, wrong worldview of his time in the early 1600s or as Martin Luther did in denouncing the corruptions of a monopolistic Roman Catholic priesthood mired in abuse of power and payoffs in the 1500's.

For many years — decades actually — the people of America have been told a series of outright lies, half truths and evasive disinformation about the subject of cancer. Combined with bad science, hidden agendas, conscious medical politics by self-interest groups determined to protect their careers, and suppression of cancer cures which worked but were made illegal, this has resulted in monstrous suffering and death for millions of people. A tragedy and a crime of monumental, historic importance rises before all of humanity now. Just as during the middle 1800's the issue of slavery suddenly, irreversibly arose in America, Russia, and other places and could no longer be ignored, so the issue of medical tyranny, especially in cancer treatment, now emerges full-blown for people alive now to face and end.

At the heart of the issue, tragically, is bad science. This may be the saddest aspect. As this book will describe in very clear language, defying orthodox science's lies and orthodox science's muscle, standards and principles of science have been perverted in order to keep an "old guard" in power and maintain its scientific illusions. Abuse of scientific procedures by politicized "old boy" networks, rigid control of research funds, bureaucratic obstacle courses designed to obstruct or prevent innovative science and healing from being delivered to patients, and many other crude or sophisticated evil practices by scientists, doctors and government health officials have been employed. What was the result? Again, terrible tragedy was repeated millions and millions of times in countless homes for families who were absolutely ignorant of how a few powerful men (and women) belonging to a medical-scientific class or elite, professional "tribe" destroyed so many innocent lives. It is not a pretty picture, you will discover in this book, but it will be all laid out for you the reader to examine and assess. Future reformers and historians will have great amounts of documentary evidence to deliver the judgment of time.

That is why now is a revolutionary turning point which begins the end of a monstrous, invisible, medical tyranny. The next decade will witness scores of new Rife-related or Rife-inspired energy medicine breakthroughs, discoveries and inventions. Simultaneously, the evil medical politics of decades will be exposed widely to future generations. Hopefully, new constitutional protections will be put in place for the individual citizen in order that medical evil, such as has existed, will never, never be allowed again.

CHAPTER 3:
A FEW OUTRAGEOUS SUPPRESSIONS SUMMARIZED (TO GET THE ANGER JUICES FLOWING)

There has never been admission or acknowledgment of the great medical crimes which have occurred again and again. Some of these crimes will be briefly summarized in this chapter but, again emphasized, because the medical officials, decade after decade, have buried or covered up the most serious crimes, the average citizen and the elected officials who represent the people have not taken steps — enacting laws and procedures — which would prevent or at least provide protections against similar crimes being perpetrated in the future. Sweeping these terrible misdeeds under the rug enables the same kind of dirty medical politics to happen again and again. This fundamental failure must be recognized if a permanent, lasting antidote to the current evil is to be created.

So, let us review together the record of the cancer atrocities which have never been acknowledged openly to the average citizen so that the average citizen can be on guard. That is one purpose of insisting that the medical moguls own up to what they or their predecessors did, with the result being (a) a perversion of the underlying principles which are supposed to govern medicine and science; (b) a tyrannical usurpation of political rights and protections which are the average citizen's constitutionally protected, legitimate expectation; (c) suffering and death for millions.

In reviewing a few of the most blatant and egregious acts against the American people, let us begin with the American Medical Association (AMA).

Morris Fishbein reigned supreme as the medical dictator of America in the 1930's and 1940's. Elevated to his position as head of the

American Medical Association in 1924 when his predecessor was found guilty in a court of law of malicious, criminal acts against his wife, Fishbein slowly consolidated his power during the second half of the 1920's decade. By the early 1930's however, he began a 20 year reign of tyranny and suppression of alternative healing which reverberates monstrously into modern times. In many ways current policies and practices of the AMA continue a direction established by Fishbein.

Fishbein appeared on the cover of *TIME* magazine, challenged (and defeated) President of the United States Franklin Roosevelt on national health issues, and openly, vehemently attacked electronic healing therapies for no other reason than they threatened the wallets and bank accounts of the AMA doctors.
Fishbein admitted that the public health be damned. His job was to protect the financial interests of AMA doctors:

> *"How is the individual physician who knows little or nothing of the physical basis of electricity and, in fact, who knows little or nothing of any physics at all.., to have any actual knowledge of these modalities?"*
>
> *"The introduction of unknown forces into the treatment of disease meant that physicians untrained in the basic sciences on which a comprehension of these forces depends must begin anew their period of infancy and education, or yield their patients and their livelihood to those better informed."* (1)

"Or yield their patients." Fishbein's blatant, openly admitted motives for all the reprehensible deeds which he and his AMA committed against alternative forms of healing and the American people — greed and power.

Fishbein's AMA was a cesspool of drug kickbacks, promotion of dangerous products where he had a financial interest, and behind-the-scenes political acts to destroy anyone who challenged his dictatorial whims and financial schemes.

Harry Hoxsey and William Koch were two of the better known individuals with respected cancer therapies who were viciously destroyed by Fishbein's mad, evil delusions and absolutist power urges. Hoxsey had refused to sell an effective cancer herbal treatment to Fishbein and his AMA cronies. Koch similarly challenged Fishbein's absolutism. They and the American people soon paid the price of incurring Fishbein's wrath. The cost to cancer patients for decades to come was, of course, torture and death because these unique approaches to treating cancer were stomped by Fishbein's megalomania.

A series of court actions, thuggery, and attempted murder were employed to prevent Dr. Koch's cancer cure from reaching mainstream America. Doctors who successfully used the drug to cure cancer lost their hospital privileges. A few doctors who supported Dr. Koch lost their lives under mysterious circumstances.

> *"(There was) one death from poisoning and one from being run down by an automobile, both victims being prominent in the advocacy of of the Koch treatment. Mail has been opened and Dr. Koch himself was the target of at least 13 unsuccessful attempts on his life."* (2)

Royal R. Rife, the quiet genius working in his San Diego laboratory with his great microscope invention, his electronic healing, his successful cancer clinics, and his brilliant scientific discoveries relating to the dwarf bacteria or virus-size microbes associated with cancer and other diseases, was another victim of Fishbein and the AMA. When the local San Diego Medical Society attacked Rife and the doctors who were using Rife's incredible futuristic electronic instruments, the climate created by Fishbein and his American Medical Association certainly was a factor. Circumstantial evidence suggests Fishbein's role probably was much, much more hands on in directing the suppression of Rife but — to be careful at this distance in time — let us merely note that Fishbein was actively, consciously involved in destroying the threat of electronic healing. That is absolutely certain and documented. Fishbein wrote and spoke about his aim and intention openly and often. And Fishbein and the AMA succeeded in their terrible betrayal of the American people and the public trust. At least until the 1990's brought the big revival of energy medicine and many other alternative healing therapies.

The electronic healing association which opposed the AMA in the 1930's was a national organization with thousands of members, many of whom were medical doctors. It was wiped off the map by Fishbein's and the AMA's vicious, criminally illegal campaign. They got away with not just commercial crime but mass murder. By the 1950's, the electronic healing association was extinct! It was Fishbein's dreadful legacy. He was sort of an American Torquemada or Grand Inquisitor of Medicine, ultimately responsible for torturing and destroying millions and millions of people. As with the Spanish Inquisition centuries earlier, Fishbein — like Torquemada — initiated a bloodbath of historic proportions. History will record Fishbein's infamy. As the noted author C. S. Lewis once observed:

> *"The greatest evil is done in clean, carpeted, warmed and well-lighted offices by quiet men with white collars."*

The AMA was and, to some extent, still is today an organized syndicate which secretly, and not so secretly, spied on and destroyed all rivals to its monopoly, using price-fixing, payoffs, media censorship and a public relations "800 pound gorilla" approach in eclipsing various alternative therapies, not to mention the ruthless criminal dark side — labs mysteriously burned, doctors who advocated alternatives beaten by thugs, and so forth. The American public never has learned how their individual personal health was adversely affected by dirty AMA decisions and policies in "well lighted offices by quiet men with white collars."

In the 1950's, after Fishbein left the AMA, his culture continued to produce evil actors performing familiar outrages. An awesomely effective cancer therapy called Krebiozen came onto the scene. Championed by Dr. Andrew Ivy, Vice-President of the University of Chicago and certainly one of the most renowned cancer researchers of his time, Krebiozen eventually was used by thousands of doctors on thousands of cancer patients. The results were remarkable.

Unfortunately, such results didn't matter very much because the Treasurer of the AMA, J. J. Moore, decided arbitrarily that two of his business cronies (with almost certainly a slice for himself) ought to have ownership of this important cancer therapy. Moore bragged to several people that if he didn't get ownership, he'd destroy Krebiozen, no matter how effective it was. Dr. Ivy and the men who discovered Krebiozen refused to sell it to the AMA Treasurer's front men so, the AMA Treasurer took his revenge. Reaching into the highest levels of the United States government's health bureaucracy (the National Cancer Institute and the Food and Drug Administration), J. J. Moore destroyed Krebiozen merely because he couldn't obtain ownership. Witnesses testified under oath before the Illinois state legislature regarding the AMA Treasurer's statements and threats. No matter. Powerful forces had arranged that the legislative inquiry would be limited. Therefore, despite the accusations, the AMA's J. J. Moore never had to testify under oath himself! It was a blatant political cover-up of the AMA's Treasurer caught in an old AMA arm twisting scheme. The result was predictable. The AMA got away with murder — mass murder. Krebiozen was totally suppressed.

The United States Senator from Illinois, Paul Douglas, later commented that it was a sad thing that Americans could no longer trust the NCI or the FDA. It was a prophetic remark. Time would eventually demonstrate just how corrupt and tyrannical both government agencies (the NCI and the FDA) would become.

As for the AMA's role in suppressing Krebiozen, Senator Douglas stated on a David Wolper TV documentary in the 1960's:

"The medical politicians do not like innovation. There

> *are a lot of other circumstances in this Krebiozen case which may implicate the American Medical Association itself."* (3)

As early as 1953, a United States Senate report concluded:

> *"There is reason to believe that the AMA has been hasty, capricious, arbitrary, and outright dishonest. Krebiozen is one of the most promising materials yet isolated for the management of cancer. I have gone over the records of 530 cases by unbiased cancer experts and clinics. I have concluded that in the value of present cancer research, this substance and the theory behind it deserves the most full and complete and scientific study. Behind and over all this is the weirdest conglomeration of corrupt motives, intrigue, selfishness, jealousy, obstruction and conspiracy that I have ever seen. Public and private funds have been thrown around like confetti at a country fair to close up and destroy clinics, hospitals, and scientific research laboratories which do not conform to the viewpoint of the medical associations. We are under a compelling moral obligation to the untold millions of cancer sufferers throughout the world to carry on this investigation. We cannot do otherwise."* (4)

The United States Senate report made no difference. Krebiozen was totally suppressed. The AMA was not investigated. It continued on the corrupt course established by Fishbein. But then one courageous chiropractor, assisted by one courageous attorney, stood up to the AMA. It may have started something which will, in time, end the AMA's evil acts.

Chiropractic was invented in 1895 and by the late 1990's was used by 20 million Americans. There currently exist approximately 55,000 chiropractic practitioners in the United States. (5)

Chester A. Wilk, the chiropractor, started his law suit against the AMA on October 2, 1976. His attorney was George McAndrews, assisted by Paul Slater and others. All deserve the gratitude of millions of Americans now living and countless more belonging to future generations who have not yet been born.

In the course of a 13 year and 4 month struggle which ended on Feb 7, 1990 with the federal conviction of the AMA, Chester A. Wilk and his attorneys discovered that H. Doyl Taylor, Director of the AMA's Department of Investigation, was the individual directing a nationwide conspiracy against chiropractic. The stated goal, introduced into the court records in the form of an AMA document, was *"ultimately the elimination of chiropractic."* Just as the AMA had done in Fishbein's time in destroying legitimate, effective, scientifically-based cures for cancer.

When it was time to call the AMA's H. Doyl Taylor as a witness in the trial, under oath, what happened? He ran to avoid testifying just as the AMA's J. J. Moore had managed to avoid testifying under oath in the Krebiozen legislative hearings.

Chester A. Wilk, the courageous chiropractor, later asked, *"What kind of person would devote his life to such dishonesty?"* (6)

Finally, through the long process of appeals, the AMA's H. Doyl Taylor was forced to testify on videotape from the distant state to which he had moved in order to avoid telling the incriminating facts concerning the AMA's conspiracy.

Also, critically in the second trial, an AMA document from a member of the AMA's Board of Trustees to the AMA's chief lawyer, clearly revealed that findings for over 40 years had shown that chiropractic was effective! The AMA had decided to lie to the American people instead of cooperating to end pain and suffering for millions and millions of trusting folks. Fishbein's continuing legacy!

The United States Court of Appeals for the Seventh Circuit ruled on February 7, 1990 in the great AMA conspiracy case. That ruling serves as a great light which touches glowingly many, many other alternative healing approaches. The Court declared:

> *"Relief here is provided not only to the plaintiff chiropractors, but also in a sense to all consumers of health-care services. Ensuring that medical physicians and hospitals are free to professionally associate with chiropractors likely will eliminate such anticompetitive effects of the boycott as interfering with consumers' free choice in choosing a product (health care provider) of their liking. In this way, competition is served."* (7)

Chester A. Wilk's precise wording explains the great importance of his victory over the AMA monster:

> *"With over 57,000 members worldwide, chiropractic is the largest drug-free health profession in the world."*
> *"For decades, unnoticed and unhindered, the orthodox medical establishment has limited our right to choose among the various approaches to health care. We have been programmed to think of health care as consisting of drugs and surgery."* (8)

During a 1997 radio interview, Chester A. Wilk declared:

> *"If there is ever an organization that deserves a Congressional investigation for dishonesty and fraud, in my opinion, it is the American Medical Association."* (9)

Amen!

> *"For most of this century, the American Medical Association deemed it unethical for physicians to refer patients to chiropractors, or the 'unscientific cult.' Now, medical researchers are conceding that chiropractors can offer relief for lower back pain."* U.S. News & World Report, (October 11, 1999), p.68

CHAPTER 4: MEDIA MUSCLE AND BIASED SCIENCE EQUALS? (ANSWER: CENSORSHIP AND FIFTH RATE SCIENCE.)

Money, power and vast public relations networks which drown out competing medical voices — Welcome to the world of the AMA's "800 pound gorilla" and how local, national and international media just surrender to its size without any consideration of the effect on common people's health. This awful reality is at the center of why the American public hasn't a clue concerning the AMA's crimes and why those crimes continue to bring torture and death to so many.

The AMA public relations muscle is truly awesome:

> *"The American Medical Association press office deluged 2,500 media outlets around the world with press packets, E-mails, faxes and, for broadcasters, tantalizing chunks of ready-to-air film footage. JAMA (Journal of the American Medical Association) licenses 15 international editions and circulates to 750,000 readers in 150 countries. 'JAMA Report,' a two-and-a-half minute 'video news release' accessible via satellite to every television network and local station in the country, reaches an average of 25 million and as many as 110 million viewers see at least part of it every week."* (10)

It's all a business of course, masquerading as science and medicine, and since the AMA depends — as it has for decades — on drug company advertisements, anything related to natural therapies is, well, contained in rigid, mental boxes and often questionable "scientific" studies. As two reporters from the Chicago Sun Times, which is physically located just one block from the AMA headquarters, described the drug company / AMA "marriage" in dollars:

"scientific" studies. As two reporters from the Chicago Sun Times, which is physically located just one block from the AMA headquarters, described the drug company / AMA "marriage" in dollars:

> *"The AMA already is hooked on pharmaceutical company advertising, which makes up about 20 percent of its operating revenue, second only to members' dues, as a source of AMA funding."* (11)

It all simply means that America's scientific and medical system is now hopelessly corrupt. Billions of dollars in research funds and approved medicines — excluding, of course, alternative therapies and advanced energy instruments capable of near miraculous healing — are provided a public which has been brainwashed for decades. Even when alternative therapies are evaluated, who does it? People trained in orthodox medicine whose career advancement and even next week's salary require that they don't get too far out of line, that's who!

To state it again, slightly differently, so that the reader understands the issue when he or she reads in the newspaper or sees on television the latest scientific study: Can the researchers do quality science even if they dared? The answer is: rarely, in a system gone bad.

Thus medical information to the average American is controlled, subtly, and based on commercial realities, but very effectively. Again, dollars and media muscle count, not great, new, immediately workable scientific truths. These rarely get analyzed, let alone approved by the government regulators or the state medical boards.

Here, reader, are some more eye openers. May you start to see:

> *"The politics of health care are mostly nonsense and the talk of patients' rights is largely a sham. (This is) U. S. health care, the $1 trillion-plus activity that constitutes 14% of the nation's annual budget."* (12)

> *"NIH (National Institutes of Health), (is) the manager*

of the world's largest bankroll for health research: $15.6 billion this year." (13)

The proposed annual budget for the National Cancer Institute, as the decade of the 1990's closed, was $3.1 billion! That is every year! Not a dime went to Royal R. Rife's energy medicine alternative which had cured cancer 65 years earlier and had never in all that time gained the slightest curiosity of orthodox researchers and government health bureaucrats. Hmmm, isn't that odd?

Meanwhile, in the closing days of 1998, America bombed Iraq.

"One-quarter billion dollars was spent on the first night's bombing." (14)

Also, consider this. The federal budget passed in October 1998 included the following beauties while cancer patients screamed in agony and died in the thousands because of a medical-science system rotten to its core, corrupt and evil beyond words:

1) Item: $100 million for a 52 mile road in Arkansas.
2) Item: $2.5 million for the U. S. Office of Cosmetics and Color.
3) Item: $250,000 for a study of caffeinated gum.
4) Item: $250,000 for a lettuce researcher.

By the 1990's most of the orthodox medical world was hopelessly corrupted by commercial linkages. That means the researchers who obtained the massive government funds also received retainers and various kickbacks from the drug companies. As even the essentially gutless Los Angeles Times (regarding their medical reporting, especially cancer) reported:

"An ever fiercer competition for research funds, burgeoning commercialism and a growing willingness by scientists to sidestep traditional checks and balances are undermining the quality of information the public receives about advances in science and medicine. In-

creasingly, even the prestigious journals are driven by market forces rather than scientific ones." (15)

The end result of this is bad science, restricted to safe, orthodox channels, and dreadful options for the cancer patient. A vast system of cancer hospitals and a monopoly on cancer therapies are controlled by surgeons, radiologists and "chemo-nuts." No one else really gets to participate on the cancer wards. Whose rights are thus denied? — The cancer patient, obviously.

When one of the leading cancer doctors in the country admits openly that he gave cancer patients chemotherapy which he knew would not help them because he wanted to prevent them from trying alternative therapies, actual madness exists and is parading in the doctor's priest-like white coat. Charles G. Moertel of the prestigious Mayo Clinic did exactly that. Moertel is now dead but he was an awesome power in cancer medicine well into the late 1990's.

Moertel's admission should never be forgotten in light of the 10,000 Americans who die of cancer every week.

> *"After Moertel took the patients in his (1985) study off vitamin C, he put most of them on a powerful chemotherapeutic drug that he had acknowledged in scientific publications to be unable to 'produce benefit or extension of survival.' I couldn't understand why Moertel would give toxic drugs he knew would not help them, until I saw a remarkable paper he published."* (16)

Moertel's paper stated:

> *"Patients have a compelling need for a basis of hope. If such hope is not offered, they will quickly seek it from the hands of quacks and charlatans."* (17)

So Moertel decided it would be better that his cancer patients died with Moertel's useless chemotherapy than be allowed precious time to investigate and possibly experiment with alternative therapies that sometimes actually cured cancer. Moertel and the Mayo Clinic had gone way over the ethical line and the physician's obligation, both morally and legally. They were playing God.

But let us briefly return to the media role. No hard information gets out regarding alternative cancer therapies to mainstream Americans. The AMA and the drug companies control what most Americans read in their mainstream newspapers and on the national networks.

Here is former Surgeon General Everett C. Koop bravely blasting ABC Nightly News for its biased medical coverage:

> *"'You don't find Peter Jennings quoting anything else in his newscasts,' Koop says. 'It's the New England Journal (of Medicine), JAMA (Journal of the AMA) or nothing.'"* (18)

In the late 1980's and early 1990's, a Los Angeles chiropractor named Gary L. Glum began telling Americans about four herbs which had successfully worked on cancer for decades in Canada. President John F. Kennedy's own physician eventually became involved and enthusiastically promoted the now familiar Essiac. But Glum was the person who truly, courageously pushed it into the natural health crowd's awareness. At one point in time, he approached the ABC News executive producer. Here's what happened:

> *"We took it to Joe Donally who's the executive news producer for ABC in New York. He said, 'Nope.' He went on to say he's got a mortgage on his house and he's looking forward to retirement. So that's the problem. No one wants the information disseminated."* (19)

Ten thousand Americans die from cancer every week, week after week, month after month, but the doctors, researchers, government health officials, media, elected representatives and senators of the United States Congress mostly turn away. It's a blasphemous crime. Compare it to an ongoing military slaughter and imagine how quickly the status quo would be changed at the command level with those kind of continuing losses — Overnight!

Think of the general who sends his men to take a hill. He wins the hill but loses 10,000 men. Then the hill is evacuated a week later. It doesn't require a military genius to realize that a week later or a year later or ten years later the "victory" for that hill may be viewed as a total defeat. 10,000 men lost for what later may be determined as a worthless piece of real estate.

A general who did that over and over would soon be relieved of duty — permanently.

Similarly, a bureaucrat who loses 10,000 cancer patients this week and 10,000 next week, and another 10,000 the following week, on and on, while he or she is sitting on a quality cure, but playing medical politics, is criminally incompetent. America has hundreds, if not thousands of such individuals in government health agencies, key research positions, medical groups, etc. — all looking out for their own paychecks and letting 10,000 of their brothers and sisters go down while this deadly, delusional game of misplaced regulatory oversight and corrupt financial bargains continue. It's a monstrous deceit perpetrated by those unwilling to destroy an evil system which daily commits institutionalized murder.

The two Chicago Sun Times reporters who investigated the AMA made it clear that the American people could not trust their health to doctors or the AMA.

> *"We broke a series of stories in 1989-90 on financial scandals involving the AMA's top managers. We see the AMA, as more often than not, a political entity that claims to be tending to the public's health, while in reality looking after doctor's interests. However, what's good for the AMA and its members is not necessarily good for the USA."* (20)

The mainstream media keeps its lips zipped about these crimes which have gone on for decades — how unholy and immoral — beyond words, dishonest, disgusting, tragic, shameful, and inhuman.

Yet, a grassroots movement toward alternative medicine is now so powerful — and the Internet will fuel it even more — that the medical establishment is trying to regulate, control, constrict it while posturing that an evolutionary, scientific process evaluating alternative therapies is needed. It all comes down to the fact that a very great threat to orthodox medicine's dollar interest has rapidly emerged from below. The medical moguls are scrambling to contain it. Why? Is it because their carefully constructed monopoly is threatened?

> *"Four in 10 adults used alternative therapies last year, creating a $21.2 billion industry. Between 1990 and 1997, visits to alternative practitioners jumped about 47%."* (21)

The struggle to enable alternative cancer therapies into the choice equation for cancer patients remains the great battleground between the "chemo-nuts" who control the system and the 10,000 who will die every week, usually after years of torturous, unnecessary agony. The fifth rate science of the National Cancer Institute was set in stone during the 1980's by its director Vincent DeVita.

> *"Vincent 'Bulldog' DeVita (was) a mean, miserable man. He never forgot who crossed him. DeVita built his scientific reputation by pioneering in chemotherapy. He believed in 'full-dose' chemo, really aggressive treatment against cancer. These highly toxic chemicals designed to kill cancer cells often debilitated patients — a kind of full dose poison."*
>
> *"DeVita's high dose chemo became standard operating procedure at the National Cancer Institute under*

his reign." (22)

DeVita was followed as director by his protégé, Samuel Broder. The chemo madness continued. The National Cancer Institute was filled to the rafters with a tribe of "chemo-nuts."

Dr. Glenn Warner, a renowned alternative cancer physician who fought orthodox medicine's evil straitjacket therapies, succinctly defined the problem (deliberate and systematic murder by the "chemo-nuts"). Dr. Warner declared for the record of history, as a cancer physician with decades of experience, both inside and outside the cozy guild of cancer specialists:

> *"We have a multi-billion dollar industry that is killing people right and left, just for financial gain."* (23)

> *"Doctors and oncologists don't want chemotherapy to be disproved. That is where their money is."* (24)

The current medical structure of scientists, doctors and government agencies is designed to prevent individualized, alternative approaches from getting any kind of toe-hold in the world of cancer treatment. Incomes and power are threatened if this should happen! As a scholar from Australia concluded after a careful examination of the cancer cartel in America:

> *"The very organization and structure of professionally endorsed cancer research and treatment function to exclude unconventional treatments."* (25)

This is Fishbein's legacy!

CHAPTER 5: MORE MEDIA, MORE MISCHIEF, MORE UTTER MADNESS

Arnold Relman was once editor of the *New England Journal of Medicine* (*NEJM*) which is usually acknowledged as the only prestigious rival to the *Journal of the American Medical Association* (*JAMA*). In a 1992 article in the *Atlantic Monthly* journal, following his retirement from the *NEJM*, Relman confessed that society has granted a monopoly license to doctors, but that obligations accompany the monopoly. There is a great implication in this simple statement, of course, and it is one which ought to be seen as critical for the very, very important health revolution now shaping before it surges. The implication is that the doctor's monopoly may be retracted or taken back, with a different health provider structure established. It is sort of like democracy being built from the ground up following the overthrow of a tyrant or a tyrannical system in which those given power abused it and thus, could never again be entirely trusted.

Relman wrote in 1992:

> *"The highest aspiration of the medical profession... has always been to serve the needs of the sick. And that has been the basis of a de facto contract between modern society and the profession."*
>
> *"What are the terms of this contract? In this country (America), state governments grant physicians a licensed monopoly. Physicians have enjoyed a privileged position in the expectation that they will remain competent and trustworthy and will faithfully discharge the fiduciary responsibility to patients proclaimed in their*

ethical codes." (26)

Oh, oh! Competent? Doesn't that have something to do with investigating and using the latest and most effective therapies for the sake of the patient and not ignoring or stonewalling or obstructing or censoring something because it threatens their high fees and possibly obsolete knowledge? Huh?

Trustworthy? That goes to the core of doctor ethics and the sacred Hippocratic Oath which includes the following key sentence:

> *"Into whatever houses I enter, I will go into them for the benefit of the sick, and will abstain from every voluntary act of mischief and corruption."*

Of course most doctors honor the oath, but a doctor truly cannot be a member of the AMA, given its history, and totally resonate with the oath because the oath requires, as do fiduciary legal obligations, that the patient's interests far, far supersede any doctor interests. So doctors who continue to live in the AMA tent as that organization's murderous history becomes well known, must be viewed as something akin to German doctors in the concentration camps during the Nazi era. A harsh judgment, but appropriate, given the millions who have died because of AMA policies, deceit, criminal acts, and especially the organized suppression of effective cures for cancer.

> *"As a result of the medical trials at Nuremberg in 1946 and 1947, most people became aware of the medical atrocities and war crimes.., in most Nazi medical crimes.., it is likely that the chief motive was not politics or ideology but simple opportunism, self-interest, and career advancement."* (27)

So, now we are getting very close to the nub of the cancer holocaust and America's medical-scientific blasphemy or contempt for the sacred responsibilities that accompany the physician's or scientist's profession — the obligations of truth; the obligations of serving the cancer patient's interest foremost; the obligations of not becoming part of or remaining within an evil system; one's higher, personal bond or linkage with God or Spirit or Light or Higher Good, however one may define that claim or attunement.

This brings us full circle to media dishonesty and disinformation, cancer doctors' decades-long sellout of their patients, scientific betrayal of the worst kind, elected officials' political treachery and expedient sacrifice of the American people's long-term health interests. All of this complexifies, in the psychological sense of a deep blockage within the American nation and people. Complexes need to be rooted out, purged, cleansed, brought up from the dark depths of repression. This is what we now must face openly and bravely. In the years ahead, the American nation must take that hard step — one way or another. It would be best to be honest with ourselves and transform the existing scientific-medical structure. If we don't, it is likely we will be destroyed by the ongoing evil of the existing medical-scientific atrocities.

Let us be clear about the scientific situation, treachery, trickery, and fraud and the cheating, the game, the politically correct bureaucratic shuffling.

David F. Horrobin in an article published in Journal of the American Medical Association, of all places, stated bluntly and clearly that the medical science structure which now exists has failed. He even asserted the dirty little secret, one rarely discussed openly and even more rarely stated in a prominent publication, that pathological thinking is a factor in the medical scientific mess the American society now finds itself.

> *"We may just have been unlucky in that in the past thirty years the vast increases in research expenditures have not brought commensurate increases in patient care. But I think we must take seriously the possibility that we have traded innovation for quality control, not only in medical publishing but throughout medical science."*

> *"Numerous cases of scientific fraud.., have been documented.*
> *"What some call psychopathology is not rare in the scientific community."* (28)

Of course spectacular discoveries and inventions which make history rarely are accepted by the dominant scientific authorities of any given time. Professional sickness and even insane behavior patterns among ruling elites have occurred throughout history. Civilization's evolution has been long and hard. Mediocrity in science is certainly not new either, despite the arrogance of those who parade as experts.

> *"A safe generalization is that many of the scientists and much of what they publish today are mediocre at best."*
> *"Only a few scientists contribute to scientific progress. The majority publish work that has little or zero impact on the forward march of knowledge."* (29)

Royal R. Rife, of course, was one of the truly scientific geniuses of the early to middle 20th century. He was skewered by the small, mediocre minds of his time. He threatened their prestige and their incomes, so they destroyed him even though the cost in human lives was staggering.

It is, perhaps, time for the outsider geniuses to be allowed their chance in vital areas of science and medicine. The credentialed experts who have been hogging all the dough and the spotlight have failed over and over in the cancer ward. The outsiders just may show us the way clear from the deadly commercial science and political medicine which threatens American society and the world as surely as the Soviet Union's tyranny did in its menacing heyday. The parallel is apt. We ignore it at our peril.

President Dwight D. Eisenhower warned future generations, in his famous farewell address of 1961, that government grants, combined with arrogant experts, could destroy both democratic values and intellectual truth-seeking.

> *"Partly because of the huge costs involved, a Government contract becomes virtually a substitute for intellectual curiosity."*
> *"The prospect of domination of the nation's scholars by Federal employment, project allocations and the power of money is ever present, and is gravely to be regarded."*
> *"We must be alert to the danger that public policy could itself become the captive of a scientific-technological elite.*
> *"It is the task of statesmanship to integrate these forces within the principles of our democratic system."* (30)

With President Eisenhower's wisdom and strength as a guide, let us return to Arnold Relman who opened this chapter with his admission that doctors had been given a monopoly in return for certain actions on their part. Then, let us examine Relman's own behavior in light of President Eisenhower's admonition or even warning concerning "a scientific-technological elite." Finally, let us place the issue in the larger context of the terrible history of medical malice in cancer treatment, as described in preceding chapters.

What do we find? Arnold Relman and his live-in lady friend Marcia Angell, current executive editor of the <u>New England Journal of Medicine</u>, together are involved in a furious, elitist attack against alternative medicine. All the while the <u>NEJM</u> continues to accept millions of dollars each year from the drug companies. What a quaint coincidence.

> *"<u>The Lancet</u> (respected British medical journal) referred* to the <u>NEJM</u> *as 'a competitive business not an altruistic academic enterprise.' It points out that 'the*

> *NEJM is nothing if not a successful business — at least $19 million in display advertising sales accrue to the journal each year.' The majority of those funds come from the pharmaceutical industry."* (31)

Now don't forget those 10,000 lives sacrificed to cancer every week, while the cute elites play intellectual games and keep the walls erected against objectively testing the alternative therapies for cancer.

But let us briefly return to the Journal of the AMA before completing the tale of Relman and his New England Journal of Medicine live-in pal.

In 1998, the Journal of the AMA (JAMA) sought to take a neutral position on alternative healing. JAMA had been under the direction of George Lundberg since the early 1980's (and thus he was long tainted by the AMA's untruthful public posturing during the 1980's struggle with the chiropractors which ended in a federal conviction of the AMA for conspiracy). Thus it was not surprising that JAMA's new, "neutral" position regarding alternative medicine was viewed by people familiar with the AMA's long, corrupt history to be little more than smoke and mirrors. Still, compared to the New England Journal of Medicine's mindless, biased attacks against alternative healing, the AMA seemed almost reasonable. Almost.

JAMA's "little" opening to alternative healing was primarily focused on the soft, essentially non-doctor threatening aspects, such as herbs. The big, dangerous, taboo regions such as energy medicine which directly threatened the drug company empires remained beyond discussion. The AMA definitely did not want the suppression of a cure for cancer 65 years earlier followed by the suppression of the entire field of electronic healing (and all the lost, related science) of 50 years earlier laid at its doorstep. The American public might be very unhappy with that revelation.

So the relatively safe subject of herbs was permitted into an occasional article in JAMA. The AMA medical politicians had skillfully managed such threats to their monopoly previously and there was this darn grassroots healing movement which was obviously affecting the incomes of the doctors. A $21 billion annual market (and still growing) was not something the AMA was going to ignore. The elites at the NEJM might turn their noses up at the American people's common sense (shades of Tom Paine in the Revolutionary War) but the AMA saw market forces and tons of dollars. Thus "neutrality" to the softer aspects of alternative healing appeared to be a skillful maneuver by JAMA editor Lundberg.

In March 1998, JAMA published an article by Wayne Jonas, at the time the Director of the Office of Alternative Medicine. It parroted the AMA party line lovingly and fawningly:

> *"Patients may be putting themselves at risk by their use of these treatments. Only fully competent and licensed practitioners can help patients avoid such inappropriate use."* (32)

This was such sweet music to the AMA's long corrupt ears.

Then in November 1998, JAMA published a special issue on alternative healing with an emphasis on guess what? — Herbs! — nice and safe. Meanwhile 10,000 more cancer patients died in America that week (and 40,000 that month) while the doctor "chemo-nuts" kept pumping in their poison and raking in high fees for their talented services.

Here's a glimpse at what JAMA was up to (note the continuation of its war against chiropractic despite a federal court injunction to cease and desist):

> *"The findings of the six studies presented in the special JAMA issue range from evidence that burning an herb over a pregnant woman's foot may correct a breech presentation to research showing that spinal manipulation doesn't alleviate tension headaches."*(21)

Unfortunately for JAMA editor George Lundberg, despite his sophisticated maneuvering on behalf of the doctor monopoly, even such a small opening to the alternative health world was not appreciated by other "old dogs" of the AMA. When, in January 1999, during the height of the President Clinton-Monica Lewinsky sex scandal, JAMA editor George Lundberg published an old (1991) survey on sexual attitudes among college students, the "old dogs" saw their chance. Lundberg, despite his 18 years of service, was summarily bounced.

> *"Dr. George D. Lundberg, 65, was bounced for 'inappropriately and inexcusably interjecting JAMA into the middle of a debate that has nothing to do with science or medicine,' said AMA Executive Vice President E. Ratcliffe."* (33)

Meanwhile, at JAMA's publishing competitor, the New England Journal of Medicine, the three elites (Editor in Chief emeritus Arnold S. Relman, his live-in lady friend, executive editor Marcia Angell, and editor Jerome P. Kassirer) carried on their own private war against alternative medicine. (34)

All the while $19 million a year (coincidentally, conveniently) of drug company money rolled into the NEJM bank accounts and 40,000 Americans died of cancer every month as the "chemo-nut" doctors kept pumping the synthetic drugs into the trusting patients.

"*Snake oil*," screeched Marcia Angell of the NEJM at all alternative medicine.

The very courageous physician Julian Whitaker, whose newsletter Health and Healing reaches over 500,000 eager subscribers and readers, provides a good perspective on the three elites at the NEJM. Whitaker writes:

> *"Drs. Marcia Angell and Jerome P. Kassirer perpetuate the war against natural therapies by questioning the safety of herbs. Of course, they don't mention the 180,000 documented deaths and 1,000,000 injuries attributed to adverse reactions to prescription drugs every year. Instead they*

focus on two patients who were hospitalized for side effects of an obscure herbal preparation. Folks, this is nothing more than propaganda in the ongoing turf war of the pharmaceutical industry against natural substances they can neither patent nor control."

"It's permissible that 80% of the drugs given to children have never been determined appropriate for pediatric use?" (35)

President of the United States Dwight Eisenhower was once President of Columbia University. It was during his years at Columbia that Eisenhower developed a deep distrust of academic elites. Eisenhower left some words of wisdom for the people of America which relate to the antics of Angell, Relman and Kassirer at the NEJM as these three elites continue to rail against alternative healing.

While addressing a Joint session of the Brazilian Congress in February 1960, President Eisenhower gave the following civic lesson and guiding policy statement of a liberty-loving republic:

> *"Here is the key to our policy — the right to choose. Human beings everywhere simply as an inalienable right of birth, should have freedom to choose their guiding philosophy, their form of government, their methods of progress."* (36)

At other times and in other places, while President of the United States or serving his country in other ways, Dwight Eisenhower reminded the American people — those of his own time and also future generations, including those now living and reading these words for the first time — that they carried sacred obligations.

> *"The right of the individual to elect freely the manner of his care in illness must be preserved."* (37)

He was also crucially aware of the *"struggle between free and slave societies going on for some 3,000 years.*" (38)

But those words must now be directed to a new enemy and a new war. The "chemo-nuts" and the drug companies murder 10,000 Americans per week, as even a former President of the American Chemical Society clearly saw:

> *"As a chemist trained to interpret data, it is incomprehensible to me that physicians can ignore the clear evidence that chemotherapy does much, much more harm than good."* (39)

The American Chemical Society is no small, obscure organization. It has an "*$85 million-a-year publications division, which prints 27 journals of its own.*" (15)

John Cairns, noted cancer scholar, stated the awful truth in Scientific American in 1985. The "chemo-nuts" ignored him and just kept on pumping the poison. Cairns wrote in the prestigious journal:

> *"It is not possible to detect any sudden change in death rates for any of the major cancers that could be credited to chemotherapy. Those who organized cancer centers and supervise the many clinical trials look for ways to circumvent these relentless statistics. Chemotherapy treatments now avert, perhaps 2% or 3% of the deaths from cancer that occur each year in the U.S."* (40)

But the reality of the drug company dollar muscle and the years and years of brainwashing the American people keep the madness going. The market for prescription drugs and over-the-counter drugs show clearly that America today is a thoroughly addicted nation: "*Last year (1998), drug costs totaled more than $100 billion.*" (41)

In many ways, we live in days of terrible darkness. Unfortunately, the dawn of a different day may still be a while before arriving. Meanwhile, 10,000 more cancer victims will die this week, and another 10,000 next week.

The well-known doctor and author Robert C. Atkins told his huge readership the terrible truth about the medical establishment's lying, murderous activities as long ago as 1988 in his book _Dr. Atkins' Health Revolution._ The politicians, doctors, scientists, and government health officials then in power and their successors throughout the next decade ignored the truth, condemning millions of innocent Americans with cancer to torture and death. Here is the incisive, explosive condemnation of the orthodox medical experts by Dr. Atkins, words whose power and truth will ring far into the future:

> *"There have already been many cancer cures and all have been ruthlessly and systematically suppressed with a Gestapo-like thoroughness by the cancer establishment. The damage done to the body by an unsuccessful course of chemotherapy is often so great that the patient's immune system never recovers sufficiently for him to stand a fighting chance. Chemotherapy, when it has no chance, or only a remote chance, to work is at best stupid and at worst criminal."*

CHAPTER 6: NOW FOR SOME GOOD SCIENCE

The Office of Technology Assessment (OTA), which (during its existence) was supposed to provide objective scientific evaluations to Congress, carried the following in its 1990 report on Unconventional Cancer Treatments:

> *"There are, in general, no legal restrictions on a U. S. patient's right to choose a treatment for himself or herself, either in the United States or in foreign countries. However, some treatments are excluded from choice in the United States because they involve the use of unapproved substances that could only be offered illegally here."*
>
> *"It would be useful for thoughtful review of the 'freedom of choice' versus 'consumer protection' quandary in the interests of Americans with cancer."* (42)

What does this mean? It means the cancer patient has the legal right to choose any treatment he or she believes can bring a cure. However, powerful medical and scientific groups, protecting their own interests, have convinced politicians that consumers need protection (which they will be happy to provide at exorbitant prices). So, two legal principles supposedly conflict. As a result, it is argued by the political ruling class, some future, decisive court ruling, constitutional law or constitutional amendment needs to clear up this gray area. Until then, the insiders will study the problem.

The deeper, truer issue is that if good science demonstrates that cancer cures exist but bad science, promoted by various interest groups (the AMA, drug companies, status quo bureaucracies, politicians raking in campaign payoffs, outdated researchers protecting status and turf, etc.), keep good science out, then the gray area is no longer the counterfeit problem manufactured by the insiders. Corruption and monstrous criminal acts become the obvious, great wrong which must be righted, similar to the political awakening which occurred when slavery or denial of a woman's right to vote forced a fundamental change in the real world and how it actually works!

So, does good science exist showing there are non-drug, non-surgery, non-radiology cures for cancer? The answer is: Yes! A resounding Yes. Yes! Yes! Yes! There are still enormous scientific hurdles, many, many questions, and deep mysteries where the questions haven't even been framed yet, but once the bad science and cancer monopoly forces are removed from the cancer wards, millions of desperate cancer patients can begin to be healed. This has been proved by numerous people cured of cancer who have used a variety of approaches based on both good science and common sense.

In 1932, Edward Rosenow of the Mayo Clinic (when it deserved its medical prestige before the "chemo-nuts" gained control), described, in an internal document, the great scientific accomplishment of Royal R. Rife. Rosenow was reporting what his trained scientific eye had seen during three days of careful work and microscopic experimentation with Rife's historic light microscope invention. (Not electron microscope, which didn't exist in its earliest forms until 7 or 8 years later!) Rosenow declared:

> *"There can be no question of the existence of the filterable turquoise blue bodies (typhoid microbes). They are not visible by ordinary methods of illumination and magnification. Their visualization under the Rife microscope is due to the ingenious methods employed. Examination under the Rife microscope of specimens leaves no doubt of the accurate visualization by direct observation at the extremely high magnification obtained with this instrument."* (43)

In simple language, Rife's microscope had opened up a new world of science. Within two years, during the summer of 1934, Rife's clinic would cure sixteen of sixteen cancer patients diagnosed as "terminal." Tragically, Fishbein, the AMA and the San Diego Medical Society interfered with good science and stopped the scientific development of Rife's tremendous accomplishment.

The month following the July 1932 Mayo Clinic report, Rosenow's observations were announced to the top scientists of America through Science magazine, which even today remains the leading American journal for top-notch scientific discoveries. Here's a sample of what Rosenow of the Mayo Clinic wrote:

> *"Recently, I reported to the staff of the Mayo Clinic the more important observations made during three days, July 5, 6 and 7, 1932, spent in Dr. Kendall's laboratory at Northwestern University Medical School, Chicago"*
>
> *"Owing to the novel and important character of the work, each of us verified at every step the results obtained. Most observations with the Rife microscope were made at 8,000 diameters."*
>
> *"The following principles and methods were stated by Dr. Rife as being essential in order to visualize clearly the objects at this and higher magnifications by direct observation. Spherical aberration is reduced to the minimum and magnification greatly increased by using objectives in place of oculars. Proper visualization, especially of unstained objects, is obtained."* (44)

So incredible was the impact of Rife's science that even decades after Fishbein and the AMA blocked it, and before the Rife revival of the 1990's exploded, pictures of Rife's microscopes still occasionally appeared in mainstream newspapers. The San Francisco Examiner of November 19, 1988 published a photo of Rife's Universal Microscope. The newspaper had kept the photo all those years! But no newspaper article dared inform modern readers of what Rife had accomplished or the fact that even modern light microscopes of the 1990's were still stuck at 1,500X to 2,500X real magnification (depending on which expert you consult). Thus telling the world about Royal R. Rife's scientific discoveries and great inventions was still a bit dangerous, given the cancer death toll of all those decades, and the ongoing "chemo-nut" monopoly of cancer therapies.

Yet Rife's own words, describing his science, refuse to die:

> *"Microscopes were designed with a range of 5,000 to 50,000."*
>
> *"An electronic frequency to devitalize the (cancer) organism, the successful treatment of cancer, No tissue is destroyed, no pain is felt. No sensation is noticed. A tube lights up and 3 minutes later the treatment is completed. The virus or bacteria is destroyed and the body then recovers itself naturally from the toxic effect of the virus or bacteria. Several disease forms may be treated simultaneously."*
>
> *"The viruses were stained with a frequency of light." (45)*

Stained with a frequency of light — these microbes were not stained with chemical dyes (which kill them). They were not bombarded with electrons (which kill them), as required with electron microscopes. The microbes, as the Mayo Clinic's Doctor Rosenow reported in 1932 (!!), remained alive, visible at the high magnification which Rife's microscope accomplished. Because the microbes which caused or accompanied cancer and other deadly diseases are alive, Rife's electronic treatment or today's energy medicine treatment can be scientifically shown or proven to disable or destroy them, painlessly, in one's own home, without expensive doctors and hospitals. This is good science.

In the 1950s Dr. Robert Stafford of Dayton, Ohio was loaned a Rife energy instrument of that period. He used it with two dying cancer patients. The cancer was healed, as autopsies following death months later from other causes convincingly showed. In 1998, Dr. Stafford stated on video for the record of history:

> *"I still believe in it. This has given me a whole new vision of the world, having seen the effects of electro-magnetic fields. I've almost become a para-physicist. We're living in the electromagnetic fields. The stars, the radio waves are that, emanating from the heavens above. What we're seeing in the universe is duplicated in the cells. These are questions that have come to me because I've been exposed to Rife's philosophies."* (46)

At one time in the 1950's, a federal agency (probably FDA) sent an agent to "talk" with Dr. Stafford. They met for three hours. The agent wanted the Rife instrument which Dr. Stafford had. But the doctor refused to hand it over because it belonged to Rife and had only been loaned to him. Then the agent sought the research data which Dr. Stafford and a qualified researcher had conducted on rats. The research had shown a decisive effect on rats inoculated with cancer, curing many cancers and extending their lives substantially beyond the control group. According to Dr. Stafford's video testimony in 1998, these preliminary studies showed conclusively that rats infected with cancer cells and then treated with Rife's energy device were healed of cancer.

The FDA agent signed for the research documents and left with them. Two or three months later, they were returned by mail. One of the greatest cures for cancer on record was shown by scientific demonstration. The federal agency examined the documentary evidence gathered by qualified medical people. Countless American lives then, and for decades into the future, depended on what the health officials chose to do at that juncture in history.

They turned their backs, returning the research materials without even a thank you note or a cover letter. Millions and millions of Americans subsequently died of cancer or from the "bad science" therapies required by the medical monopoly for the next four decades.

As early as 1933, energy medicine was a front page story in the New York Times (before the AMA's campaign destroyed the entire scientific field for decades). The New York Times for October 9, 1933 reported on a prophetic speech given by the renowned surgeon George Crile to the American College of Surgeons. Crile predicted future physicians would be able to diagnose and treat patients before their diseases became apparent.

Here are Dr. Crile's words, reaching to modern times and far into the future:

> *"'The medical man of the future,' Dr. Crile said, 'would tune in on the living body as one does now on the ordinary radio. By listening in to the short-waves and the long-waves, transmitted by the various organs, he would hear the symphony played by the living organism and would determine the rhythms of the dance of life.'"*
>
> *"'Long before there was any outward evidence of disease, the physician-radio-engineer of the future would thus be enabled to tell by the reception of the life-waves whether they were playing a melody of health or whether they were signaling an SOS.'"* (47)

In the late 1980s, French scientist Jacques Benviniste, a laboratory head of the French National Institute of Health and Medical Research, conducted experiments which proved an energetic signature remained in a substance even when diluted to a point where orthodox science believed no chemical reaction was possible. Independent researchers in Canada, Israel and Italy verified the discovery. But the defenders of the status quo reacted furiously, claiming that the "*results had to be wrong.*" (48)

Canadian scientist Patricia Fortner, whose own work supported Benviniste, declared, "*We could be looking at a kind of phenomenon that shakes the present rules of microbiology, chemistry, physics and other sciences.*" (49)

Benviniste was right and the defenders of orthodox science, despite their shrill attacks, propaganda, incredible censorship efforts and absurd activities to discredit Benviniste (such as bringing in a magician to suggest fraud), were wrong! By the late 1990's, Benviniste was sending digital biology across continents!

> *"Digital biology is a radically new approach to biology. Life depends on signals exchanged among molecules. That molecules vibrate, we have known for decades. Every atom of every molecule and every intermolecular bond — the bridge that links the atoms — emits a group of frequencies. Around 1991, my experiments showed that we could transfer specific molecular signals by using an amplifier and electromagnetic coils. In July 1995, I recorded and replayed these signals using a multimedia computer. In the course of several thousand experiments, we have led receptors (specific to simple or complex molecules) to 'believe' that they are in the presence of their favorite molecules by playing the recorded frequencies of these molecules."*
>
> *"Biological systems function like radio sets, by coresonance. We can now understand how millions of biological molecules can communicate, something 'structural' biologists are at a loss to explain... Hence the inability of contemporary biologists to provide answers to the major pathologies at the end of the century."*
>
> *"At the present time, the only way to identify a molecule is to carry a sample, most often obtained invasively or even destructively, to a laboratory. With the digital method, we dispose of a signal which can be*

instantly transmitted and analyzed at the other end of the world by classic means of telecommunication."

"Completion of these projects would have immense consequences on medical diagnostic procedures and the agro-food industry, with huge technological and commercial impact."

"A final question: why are scientists so opposed to the evolution of science? Is it to defend their piece of turf?" (50)

Now, before the reader's imagination blasts him or her into the 21st century's obvious, coming energy medicine revolution, let us pause and return to a small room over a garage in 1929 where Royal R. Rife was showing visitors the future. The San Diego newspaper reported on the Rife phenomenon in 1929. The national magazine Popular Science did the same in 1931. Here is a sample:

> *"Rife began building his own microscopes in a laboratory fitted up in a room over the garage. In this little room, he has today more than $50,000 worth of microscopes and cameras. Most of them he built himself... Now doctors may sit at ease in comfortable chairs and watch bacteria in their native surroundings on a motion picture screen."* (51)

In 1940, Arthur Yale, M.D. of San Diego read the following to the California State Homeopathic Medical Society:

> *"For seventeen years Mr. Rife has succeeded in finding a vibratory rate which will kill the different invading organisms of the body. Having used this apparatus for almost two years, the writer has had the satisfaction of witnessing the disappearance of every malignant growth where the patient has remained under treatment, these included epitheliomas, carcinomas and*

some of undetermined origin." (52)

Rife saw in his magnificent microscope what he called a virus but today is probably not what is defined as a virus. However, there is a massive scientific argument brewing over the nature of viruses and whether they should even be defined as separate microbial structures. Let us not get involved there because it would take us into a wasteful distraction. Orthodox scientists love muddying the real issues with such exercises.

Instead, let us simply note for the sake of broad, "general reader" clarity that Rife was seeing a dwarf bacteria or a virus-size microbe and that this cancer-causing agent — which he had (1) isolated and identified, and (2) stained with light, not deadly dyes or deadly electrons — was alive. When Rife used a specific energy zapping of the microbe, it died. Over and over, the same results appeared in the microscope. That is good science.

When cancerous rats were similarly zapped, the cancers were healed. When humans with cancer were zapped, many (to be cautious and conservative) were also healed. This was reported by doctors and scientists working under the auspices of a University of Southern California Special Medical Research Committee from 1934 -1944; again reported by Dr. Arthur Yale of San Diego, as quoted above; once more observed by Dr. Robert Stafford of Dayton, Ohio in the 1950's; and eventually in the 1990's by a spreading group of energy medicine advocates (physicians, other kinds of licensed primary care practitioners, and just common folks who simply asserted their freedom and retracted the monopoly license from the "chemo-nuts," based on centuries of developing law).

But the bad science proponents insist there is nothing to this. These microbes can't cause the disease cancer, they claim. But when the orthodox scientists and doctors make such a claim, they are on very shaky ground.

In 1997 the Nobel Prize in Physiology or Medicine was awarded to Dr. Stanley B. Prusiner of the University of California at San Francisco. Prusiner had discovered prions in 1982 and traditional scientists had sneered at the claim for fifteen years, but he received the Nobel Prize! The mediocrities were wrong.

> *"Way out on an intellectual limb, Prusiner argued that prions break the most basic rules of biology. 'No one believed (the prion theory) because it went against conventional thinking.' Pruisiner showed that prions appeared to lack any genetic material. To biologists steeped in the knowledge that all disease organisms carry genetic material that guides their replication after they invade a host, that observation was roughly like discovering cars zipping along the freeway without engines."* (53)

Now let us go back to the year 1958 when Rife was describing his work and explaining that what he was seeing was the microbe of cancer. Even if the microbe wasn't a virus, his work resulted in many diseases, including cancer, being cured! Rife's own words:

> *"We have proven definitely that cancer is a virus or the filterable form and pathogenic portion of chemical constituents that produces the disease."*
>
> *"In our microscope, we produce a frequency of light that is in coordination with the chemical constituents of the virus under observation."*
>
> *"I worked a great deal with tuberculosis. I finally found an electronic frequency that would kill these, the virus of tuberculosis and the rod form. Used simultaneously, the patient gets well. If you use either frequency individually, you either kill the patient or you accomplish nothing."* (54)

What Rife was asserting in relation to tuberculosis was simplicity itself. If his energy medicine was directed only against the bacteria commonly assumed to be the cause of TB, the bacteria would die but it would release a deadly, smaller, virus-size, second TB microbe. This could kill a patient. This is why the famous Robert Koch — who discovered the TB bacteria in the 19th century — was unable to cure the disease. His approach released a deadly, smaller microbe which killed his patients. Rife zapped the large TB bacteria and the smaller, virus-size, second TB microbe simultaneously — Success!

But that was decades ago. Millions and millions of people have died of TB since then, and millions still do every year.

Rife described the virus-size cancer microbe as follows in 1933:

> *"The 'BX' (cancer microbe) is a filterable virus. It is a small ovoid (egg shaped) granule, highly plastic, and visible only with monochromatic light. The color is purple red. The X ray has no influence on the organism. The application of the oscillative ray should completely destroy the B.X. in the malignant tissue. Thus a new field is open to scientific investigators."* (55)

What emerges now, clearly, as the 20th century ends and the 21st century begins, is a profound energy medicine incorporating Royal R. Rife's discoveries into other, newer approaches and discoveries pioneered by modern scientists. The public, especially those with cancer, must be given access to this new science and new medicine without years of waiting while conventional thinkers with "old boy" government connections grab all the millions and millions of research grant dollars to study (and study and study) this matter in order to protect cancer patients. That kind of consumer protection of the cancer patient is not merely a deceitful use of the term, it often equates to bureaucratic murder (what later was termed "desk murderers" in relation to Nazi Germany).

Hopefully soon, Rife's great microscope, or at least its principles which made all his incredible science possible, will reemerge into the world, opening doors to great, lost truths.

Here is an extremely important communication from a man highly experienced in the world of microscopy, regarding his personal examination of Rife's Universal Microscope in 1997:

> *"The microscope images viewed at the meeting were beyond those in my experience, in regard to magnification, and were in my estimation around the 20,000X range. The configuration of the system was understandable by me to be innovative directly along the lines of Royal R. Rife's original work with optics. A good deal of development must occur to develop the sophistication which Mr. Rife was employing, but the basic principle of true magnification, which was embodied in the original Universal Microscope, has unquestionably been duplicated."* (56)

CHAPTER 7: PROBING THE MYSTERIES

It is imperative to realize and appreciate that late 20th century and early 21st century science is very different than the science of Rife's time. Rife's discoveries and therapies must fit into a much more complex medical science world. And where Rife's theories are flawed or only partially correct, requiring redefinition and adjustments to newly understood realities, that is part of the honest progression of science. Rife would have no problem with that.

But if complexity or bad science and conventional thinking is used to dismiss Rife, and the recorded results taking place today, which are Rife-derived or Rife-inspired, are ignored, that is unacceptable and a continuation of the cancer monopoly's crime, nothing more.

Also of great importance is for common people and especially cancer patients to be very aware that scientists, engineers, doctors and so on usually emphasize the hair-splitting technical issues or challenges. They are searching for scientific answers or new gizmos. Whether the motive is greed, ego or merely more knowledge, such a focus often ignores the primary issue. That issue is the person with cancer and whether a Rife device (or any other alternative therapy) is curing, or at least retarding effectively, the cancer. Too often even those who support Rife, or are at least open to Rife, slip into the professional attitude carried by various experts. The cancer patient, the 10,000 deaths per week just in America or the continuing torture associated with traditional cancer therapy, are all conveniently left to others.

Nevertheless, having emphasized the priority (use what cures the cancer patient even if the why is not understood!), cold language science does help the evolution and legitimizing of energy medicine.

Alan Blood of Australia provided the following in an Internet draft paper. It clarifies a few areas and thus helps the pursuit of truth:

> *"Despite the differences from other bacteria, today none of the many types of filterable bacteria are classed as virus, because they all have true cell phases which viruses do not have. Kendall and Rife's early observations of the filterable bacterial forms were not in fact viruses, but rather of mycoplasmas or of cell-wall deficient bacteria."*
>
> *"The link between the cancer microbes and human cancer is not universal as Rife and Kendall were tempted to believe. There are other possible scenarios besides mycoplasma infection which could trigger cancer."*
>
> *"Where live observation indicates pre-cancer pathology, Rife treatment may unmask the bacterial forms and T-cells, thus engendering anti-mycoplasma immune response. A reduction of mycoplasma population, particularly of the advanced phases, could eliminate the source of immunosuppression, which would be considered a major cancer risk factor. Because the emphasis is on immune response, various natural therapies... are considered necessary adjuncts to the Rife therapy."* (57)

In an overview of Rife's history and the stage of revival that existed in 1998 and 1999, a health research organization added the following to the internet explosion of information regarding Rife:

> *"It is a fair statement that Rife practically developed bioelectric medicine himself. There is a wide variation in the cost, design, and quality of the modern Rife frequency research instruments available. Costs vary from about $1200 to $3600 with price being no legitimate indicator of the technical competence in the design of the instrument or performance of the instru-*

ment."

"One day, the name of Royal Raymond Rife may ascend to its rightful place as the giant of modern medical science. Until that time, his fabulous technology remains available only to the people who have the interest to seek it out." (58)

The reader should now, from these two quotations in this chapter, begin to perceive the monumental mysteries and scientific issues surrounding energy medicine's future. There are legitimate questions concerning the microbiology which need high quality scientific investigation. There are a variety of Rife-like or Rife-inspired devices. There are also two deep, deep areas which must be included in any treatment's evaluation: the individual patient (how committed are they, how much will they change food habits, behavior, etc.) and what supporting protocol or procedure should accompany an energy medicine therapy for cancer.

As the decade of the 1990's closes, numerous "Rife" devices exist. The naive cancer patient or enthusiast hears or reads the name Rife and assumes wrongly that the name itself means an instant cure for cancer. He or she then orders a Rife device at prices varying from a few hundred dollars to thousands of dollars. If the results aren't as expected, the anti-alternative medicine old guard gloat in their conservative straitjackets and the game of endless research, lasting years, which does not disturb the "chemo-nuts'" monopoly grip on cancer therapy is allowed to go on.

Some cancer centers, aware of the rising demand by consumers and the utter failure of conventional treatment, have initiated cautious investigations into alternative medicine. One such hospital in this author's geographical vicinity is now collecting data for the next two years from cancer patients who are also using alternative therapies. How pathetically passive! It's like testing a single vitamin on thousands of volunteers for years, and then evaluating its effectiveness and safety.

It would be easy, if sufficient money and legal protection existed, to decide quickly and decisively how different, quality Rife instruments with proven records compare to each other and to standard chemotherapy. Weekly analysis of blood and hair would show, scientifically, the rapid remission of cancer if such courageous scientific experiments were initiated. Instead, the corrupt cancer world slouches along, playing it safe, permitting 10,000 Americans to die weekly and millions more people to be tortured by worthless, approved therapies politically imposed by a medical monopoly.

There is mass murder going on. It could be quickly stopped if a viable, volunteer-based alternative was merely announced! Instead, the ongoing cancer crime continues to be hidden. It continues to be disguised with clever arguments from lawyers, bureaucrats, public relations people, lobbyists and, of course, doctors and conventional scientists who are outraged when their expertise or recommendations are questioned. So the smooth talkers and the big censorships regarding cancer continue to deny what documented facts show. Billions of words and billions of dollars in payoffs of one kind or another cannot wipe out the "something" basic and testable which daily emerges from the muck of almost a century-long conspiracy.

So let us pause amidst these mysteries of life and the corrupt medical politics which keep us from experiencing health breakthroughs that are awesome to contemplate. Phenomenal healing is probably very simple to actually have once we gain access to a few keys.

As Michael Coyle has maintained, citing Guenther Enderlein's (1872—1968) research:

> *"Pathogenic microbes can be reverted to their lowest, primitive developmental stage, which can then be excreted by the body."*
>
> *"Many people have not experienced a prolonged period of natural well-being in their entire lives."*
>
> *"Antibiotics (are) a primarily anti-life approach. These 'quick fixes' have replaced long term biological approaches and preventive maintenance."*

"Among all the millions of microbes existing in nature, there are only two that should be understood to be constant companions in the human body and all mammals. These two microbes are indestructible, always existing in phases of development, and present in every cell of the body."

"From times immemorial they have accompanied all mammals with a developed symbiosis. But due to their pleomorphic nature and imbalances in the body's tissues and blood, they can become the primary causes of chronic illness in the body."

"The key to fighting cancer and other diseases successfully lies in the potential of destroying the pathogenic microorganisms and getting the body to excrete them. The microbial activity is the basis for the growth process of the tumor."

"The remedies can heal the individual at any stage in the growth process if the microbial progression is reversed." (59)

We need the good science which blood and tissue examination, combined with knowledge, confirm as constituting a healthy or an unhealthy person. We need the good science which knows how to reverse the causes of disease. But, we must not restrict our healing centers to a single approach such as changing the blood picture through reseeding at the microbe level. The energy diagnostics have their place also, especially as the "*dance of life*" and "*a melody of health*" (Dr. Crile's 1933 words) become more commonplace and as the bad science fades.

We certainly must not overlook the simple healing processes which the individual can learn and practice without any high tech equipment. Society thus must move toward creating and protecti new, individual health rights.

"Because health care decisions affect the patient more

> *directly than anyone else, the patient's choices, educated but not preempted by the doctor's expertise, should be controlling."*
>
> *"Patient autonomy should be recognized and protected as a distinct legal interest."* (60)

In 1975, an extraordinary event occurred at the National Cancer Institute (NCI). Into the main auditorium trooped eighty or ninety of the top NCI hotshots to listen to one of the world's recognized experts on the power of sunlight to heal cancer. John Ott told them how cancer had been successfully treated through such "light therapy." Six highly qualified doctors at six leading cancer research institutions were prepared to assist in developing this new approach. All that was needed was NCI funding and political support. Remember, this was an audience of 80 or 90 cancer experts who controlled the entire U. S. Government's cancer program!

Well guess what happened? They listened politely, got up, exited the auditorium, and went back to their world of chemotherapy, totally ignoring the stunning opportunity which had been placed before them! And twenty-five more years of chemotherapy, radiation and surgery were forced down the American people's throats while new generations of cancer experts rolled out of the universities and pranced onto the NCI stage. Tra-la-la!

In the 1990's, Steven A. Rosenberg, Chief of Surgery at the National Cancer Institute from the year 1974 through to the end of the century (and who knows how far beyond), admitted:

> *"We lacked the kind of understanding necessary to find a cure. We did not know enough even to know where to look for one."* (61)

Yet those who had cured cancer with a variety of approaches in the 20th century, as well as those who were doing so daily with alternative medicine, were ignored, suppressed, harassed and mocked by the experts. All this occurred while the cancer patient, whose interest was morally and legally preeminent, was prevented by regulations, laws and state associations of doctors from any radical choice which might save his or her life. The conventional science crowd held all the power switches and kept all doors of the cancer wards locked to outside influences.

Only in the 1990's, when the rumble from the grassroots shook the insiders, did they slowly pretend to be open to alternatives. But by then a lot of the people knew the insiders' medicine, despite increased public relations efforts, was hopelessly obsolete. As Paul D. Harris commented as early as 1991, foreseeing the coming revolution:

> *"The new science of chaos, wholeness and fractal mathematics is helping us to walk through the door to understanding and acceptance of 'Energy Medicine' and the realization that linear models are clearly unreliable."*
>
> *"There is five times more DDT in the cells of every person in America than we thought was safe ten years ago. There is over ten times more strontium 90 in the bones in every person in America than what we thought was safe ten years ago."*
>
> *"Energy medicine is the concept of viewing and treating the body from an energetic rather than a purely chemical perspective."* (62)

Within, or perhaps over, the entire concept of energy medicine exists centuries-old spiritual concepts which hopefully will be reestablished as the central feature of new patient rights. The instant healing and breathtaking realignments of natural healers, medicine men and medicine women, the overnight miracles of dream-inspired healing which go back to the archaic world of the Greeks and their sacred healing temples, and also those trained and talented souls who open the blocked Chi energy channels so much better understood in Asia — these are where the deeper mysteries exist. These realms hold the true keys to health, and if people are denied the absolute, protected legal right to pursue, experiment, practice and receive in these sacred regions, all the hoopla excitement of energy technologies and microbiology discoveries will fail us as surely as the "chemo-nuts" have murdered millions.

Thus we stand at the threshold of a great journey into a world where old mysteries become pathways to new technologies, new citizen rights, new healing systems, and miracles which become commonplace as more and more patients accomplish them.

A medical doctor, whose grandmother taught him about spiritual energies and how they worked in medical situations, tells us (simply):

> *"With the emergence of new and radical ideas about the nature of reality, now, more than ever, healing practitioners as well as average people need to become aware of their energetic selves."* (63)

CHAPTER 8: A SPHERE OF LIBERTY

We come now to the great issue which underlies the alternative health movement, the demand for choice in selecting cancer therapies, and the need for new legal protections which end the tyranny of self-serving experts protecting their interests. We touch now the great issue: *A Sphere of Liberty*.

In a monumental work of history titled *The Long Way to Freedom*, which describes humanity's and civilization's slow evolution to its current stage, the beautiful, soul-stirring concept and living principle of an individual's "sphere of liberty" is explained and celebrated. The book's author, James T. Shotwell (1874—1965), writes:

> *"A free society implies a society which feels that rights are secure and a government which is not afraid of freedom."*
>
> *" 'The only purpose for which power can be rightfully exercised over any member of a civilized community against his will, is to prevent harm to others. His own good, either physical or moral, is not a sufficient warrant. Over himself, over his own body and mind, the individual is sovereign.' (from John Stuart Mill, On Liberty, chap 1.)"*
>
> *" 'The firmest ground for confidence in the future is more than ever we realize that, while democracy must have its organization and control, the vital breath is individual liberty.' (Supreme Court Justice Oliver Wendell Holmes' address to both Houses of Congress.)"*
>
> *"Over against government itself there is a sphere of liberty which is to be preserved even as against the government itself. This has been safeguarded in the*

United States, not only by the Bill of Rights and the courts, but by a kind of social contract."

"The significance of the rise of modern science can be seen only in the light of this long perspective of human evolution. Almost overnight we are suddenly launched upon the second million years. We have no clear idea and can have none as to the kind of world which lies ahead, except for one fundamental fact, that mind will more and more take the place of muscle, that intelligence will more and more not only rule brute strength but replace it by other powers and forces."

"This new scientific era is not a mere passing interlude in human affairs like the splendor of Greece or the beauty of the Renaissance. It provides for its own continuance and will never stop."

"There must be freedom for the individual to experiment and to explore, to think and to express his thought. This is what is meant by democracy, not the rule of the many but rather the safeguarding of their freedom, a freedom that justifies itself by providing disciplined intelligence in its leadership and a critical, open-minded citizenship. It is worse than useless to create a vast system of international diplomacy and government if its control is to rest in the hands of those who are unfit for such high responsibilities, and that will be the case if the citizens are not alertly aware of their own interests and free to insist upon them." (64)

The proponents of chemotherapy and the medical politicians have taken from the American citizen the fundamental principle of individual liberty. This is the right, the absolute right, to decide what will be done with his or her own body. As John Stuart Mill declared in his famous work titled On Liberty, (and I paraphrase here) "*His* (the patient) *own good, either physical or moral, is not a sufficient warrant*" for doctors, health bureaucrats, scientific elites, whomever — let alone corrupt interest groups — to arrogantly assume they know what is best or that they are protecting the consumer. This fundamental principle of individual liberty, on which the United States was founded, was initially trespassed upon by medical politicians in the early part of the 20th century and, at the century's conclusion, had become an outright tyrannical imposition of arbitrary medical-scientific interference. The fundamental principle which is neatly termed "a sphere of liberty" must be reclaimed by individuals and then reestablished in governmental institutions (federal, state and local) which regulate and oversee cancer clinics and cancer wards within hospitals.

Colonel David Hackworth, one of the most decorated veterans of the Vietnam War, described in his book <u>About Face</u> the visits he made to the courtroom where the Nuremberg Trials were held after World War II. It was in this courtroom and others that hard core Nazis, doctors and bureaucratic desk murderers were convicted of crimes against humanity.

> *"The courtroom where Hess, Goering, and a score of other Nazis were tried for crimes against humanity was sealed up and preserved as a historic monument; the few times I went in there I stood in awe. It was as if the place was haunted; in the stillness I could feel the presence of the guilty, and of those courageous souls who testified against them in the hope that such crimes would never happen again."* (65)

As a result of the Nuremberg Trials, it became a principle of international law that no patient could be pressured into a medical treatment which he or she did not want.

> *"The Nuremberg Code, adopted after World War II, held that the patient 'should be so situated as to be able to exercise free power of choice, without the intervention of any element of force, fraud, deceit, duress, over-reaching or other ulterior form of constraint or coercion.'"* (66)

This is bolstered by the United States Supreme Court decision Cruzan v. *Director, Missouri Dept of Health*, June 25, 1990, with both conservative and liberal members of the court supporting the overriding principle and fundamental right that a government *"which is not afraid of freedom"* (James Shotwell's ringing phrase) would protect the individual's freedom to decide his or her own medical course of treatment. The Supreme Court ruled:

> *"The principle that a competent person has a constitutionally protected liberty interest in refusing unwanted medical treatment." (67)*

The great legal thinker and Justice Benjamin Cardoza, while on the Court of Appeals of New York, made explicit the underlying principle in 1914, long before the Nazi atrocities and their particular brand of desk murderers forced international law to focus on the individual's liberty over his or her own body. Simply put in Cardoza's eloquent, to-the-point words, this one sentence should remind every government health official to be wary when they start abusing the public trust which comes with their office:

> *"Every human being of adult years and sound mind has a right to determine what shall be done with his own body."* (68)

But what do we get from the health officials — respect for the law and the deeper, centuries-old principle of liberty guarding the individual's sovereignty over mind and body, as proclaimed in the long honored words of John Stuart Mill's *On Liberty*? We do not.

Instead, the American people got health bureaucrat and "chemonut" Vincent DeVita, Director of the National Cancer Institute throughout the 1980's, issuing an order to all cancer clinics and hospitals to shove high-dose chemotherapy — his personal specialty — into trusting, unaware cancer patients.

> *"DeVita issued a controversial recommendation to 13,000 cancer specialists in North America to give chemotherapy and surgery to all women with breast cancer, regardless of whether it had spread."* (69)

Ex-President Eisenhower thundered a warning to us all on June 1, 1961 after he retired, but we had grown forgetful:

> *"We consider it sheer arrogance to believe that people in Government know better for the people than they know for themselves."*

The medical monopoly has so corrupted even our laws in their favor that rampant tyranny now pervades the entire cancer treatment world. Sample this California law:

> *"California law 1707.1. The sale, offering for sale, holding for sale, delivering, giving away, prescribing or administering of any drug, medicine, compound or device to be used in the diagnosis, treatment, alleviation or cure of cancer is unlawful unless (1) an application with respect thereto has been approved under Section 505 of the Federal Food, Drug and Cosmetic Act or"* ... blah, blah, blah. (70)

It is unlawful? To give away a cure for cancer is unlawful?
Bureaucracies determine whether people can be cured of cancer and for decades they have forced chemotherapy, radiation and surgery on desperate cancer patients, to the exclusion of workable alternatives, despite decades of evidence that chemotherapy, radiation and surgery are failures against cancer?

> *"Bureaucracy serves to slow everything down. To a bureaucrat, what and why doesn't matter in the least as long as he can slow things down."* (71)

> *"People who spend their lives in bureaucracies were typically afraid of breaking rules. That was a sure way to get fired, and it cowed people to think of tossing their careers away."* (72)

But the hurricane in favor of alternative cancer treatment is coming and it will blow the bureaucrats and medical monopolies into oblivion!

Again, Eisenhower:

> *"Here in America we are descended in blood and spirit from revolutionaries and rebels. As their heirs, may we never confuse honest dissent with disloyal subversion.., through knowledge and understanding, we will drive from the temple of freedom all who seek to establish over us thought control."* (73)

The lawyers are beginning to hear and sense the sound of the coming force. The medical monopoly's twisting of law to serve their own interest is beginning to stir widespread, mainstream, citizen revolt.

> *"American allopathic physicians, along with their trade association the AMA, have attempted to define medical reality, dominate traditional non-physician practitioners and monopolize the control of health care generally."*
>
> *"A growing number of people are agitating for the right of patients to choose their own forms of medical treatment. Complex legal issues involving constitutional and antitrust law with regard to treatment choice abound."* (74)

The fundamental principle at issue remains firm, solid and absolutely unyielding. No notion of consumer protection by bureaucrats, arrogant scientists or medical unions can alter it: The sovereignty of the individual over his or her mind and body.

> *"It is now a well-established rule of general law, as binding upon the government as it is upon the medical profession at large, that it is the patient, not the physician, who ultimately decides if treatment — any treatment — is to be given at all. The rule has never been qualified in its application by either the nature or purpose of the treatment, or the gravity of acceding to or foregoing it."* (75)

The doctors, the AMA, the FDA, and the NCI must step back!

> *"Conflict of interest undermines the doctors claim to authority (and) courts may identify and protect patient choice."* (76)

It is likely that history will judge harshly these organizations and groups which so abused their power, torturing and killing so many millions.

> *"Western doctors, largely ignoring the contributions of complementary philosophies, will probably be seen in several centuries' time as being akin to the ptolemaic view that the earth was the center of the universe."* (77)

Now new sciences emerge. The clear evidence of how cancer can be cured will become part of future court records. The "chemo-nuts" will be banished from the hospitals and cancer clinics of the future.

> *"The expression 'scientific revolution' or 'revolution in science,' implies a break in continuity, the establishment of a new order that has severed its links with the past, a sharply defined plane of cleavage between what*

is old and familiar and what is new and different." (78)

James DeMeo, in a 1998 Internet newsletter release, explained how the FDA is still defying Supreme Court rulings, the law of the land:

> *"Does the FDA have the legal right to keep Americans from learning about views contrary to its own? The FDA says yes, but the Supreme Court says no. With their proposed new rules, the FDA has defied the Supreme Court decision in a case called Daubert v. Merrill Dow. Daubert replaced the 'General Acceptance Test' (an equivalent phrase to 'significant scientific agreement') with the Federal Rules of Evidence for admitting scientific testimony at a federal trial. The new standard mandated by the Supreme Court demands that there be 'significant scientific evidence' to support a claim, instead of the 'significant scientific agreement' proposed by the FDA. The difference between the two standards is enormous. The Supreme Court standard relies on scientific evidence rather than the opinions of FDA scientists and bureaucrats, who may be unaware of the evidence in favor of a claim, or may choose to ignore this evidence."* (79)

So, now the new medicine emerges with the American nation's laws in place, ready to accept the scientific evidence. A revolution is about to happen. Millions of people who develop cancer in the future will be cured rapidly by methods now available which the medical monopoly and their health bureaucracy cronies criminally denied cancer patients of the past:

> *"It is a well-established fact that one of the most important genetically encoded programs in humans is the ability to heal ourselves. Healing begins in the deepest parts of our beings — the emotional, mental*

levels — and then spreads outward to the physical level." (80)

"If science concentrated on cleansing the blood and allowing the blood to do its job of attacking cancer cells, the 'War on Cancer' could be easily won."

"When you have cancer, your whole body needs a massive overhaul. Nearly every single organ is run down and toxic: your kidneys, your liver, your colon, and your immune system. When you do the job right, and heal your entire body, the cancer will be gone for good." (81)

"Cancer is a process of progressive degeneration where cells no longer maintain a normal aerobic metabolism or a high degree of differentiation. In order to stabilize and eliminate the disease, actively promoting health through changes and lifestyle patterns makes logical sense. A specific program to both address cancer and support health might include the following four features: 1) Enhance the metabolism. 2) Cleanse the blood to take the burden off the immune system. 3) Induce the immune system to eliminate abnormal cells. 4) Normalize DNA expression." (82)

The Hippocratic Oath, the sacred oath which every doctor takes upon becoming a doctor, will be viewed seriously again in the future. The "chemo-nuts" will be asked why they did not honor it and why they gave poison to their patients. The Hippocratic Oath includes the following:

"I will use treatment to help the sick. I will never use it to injure them or wrong them. I will not give poison to anyone." (83)

All doctors who once were part of the AMA ought to be asked why they silently permitted the AMA bosses to carry on such crimes against the American public as have been shown in court testimony, documented records and decisive court decisions which declared the AMA had conducted a conspiracy. How do doctors live with themselves and continue to support such an organization?

It's a big question and it deserves a revolutionary response by doctors. Not just a cleansing of the stench within their own stables, but an open welcoming of alternative practitioners in the task of healing innocent, trusting patients who are in pain and agony.

Supreme Court Chief Justice William Rehnquist, a conservative, and Supreme Court Associate Justice William Brennan, a liberal, close this book with their shared, ringing declarations concerning the individual's "sphere of liberty" in its medical aspect. Chief Justice William Rehnquist, 1990:

> *"(No) right is held more sacred, or is more carefully guarded, by the common law, than the right of every individual to the possession and control of his own person. Justice Cardoza aptly described this doctrine: 'Every human being of adult years and sound mind has a right to determine what shall be done with his own body."* (84)

Associate Justice William Brennan, 1990:

> *"Fundamental rights 'are protected not only against heavy-handed frontal attacks, but also from being stifled by more subtle governmental interference.' 'The root premise' of informed consent is that every human being of adult years and sound mind has a right to determine what shall be done with his own body."* (85)

APPENDICES

The Courtroom

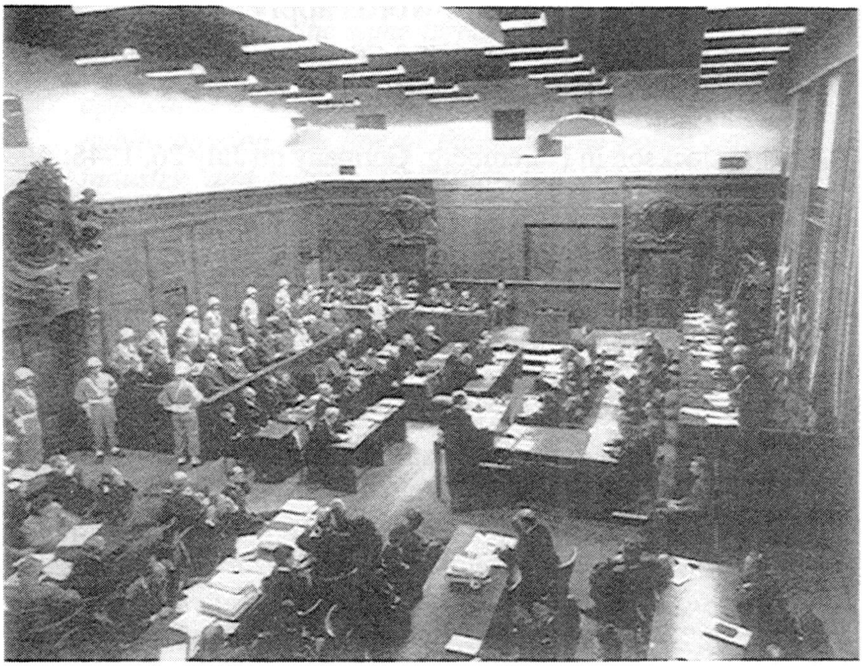

First Nuremberg Trial

APPENDIX A: SELECTIONS FROM THE AMERICAN PROSECUTOR'S SUMMATION AT THE FIRST NUREMBERG TRIAL July 26, 1946

***Some of these historic words apply to the medical-scientific crimes in America described in this book.

Robert H. Jackson in Nuremberg, Germany on July 26, 1946:

"It is impossible in summation to do more than outline with bold strokes the vitals of this trial's mad and melancholy record, which will live as the historical text of the twentieth century's shame and depravity."

"It is not their thoughts, it is their overt acts which we charge to be crimes. Their creed and teachings are important only as evidence of motive, purpose, knowledge, and intent."

"In summation, we now have before us the tested evidences of criminality and have heard the flimsy excuses and paltry evasions of the defendants... if the case I present seems hard and uncompromising, it is because the evidence makes it so."

"I put before you only the bold outlines of a case that is impressive in its simplicity. I must leave it to experts to comb the evidence and write volumes on their specialties, while I picture in broad strokes the offenses whose acceptance as lawful would threaten the continuity of civilization."

"The charge requires examination of a criminal pol-

icy, not of a multitude of isolated, unplanned, or disputed crimes.

"Laws were created of such ambiguity that they could be used to punish almost any innocent act. (Reminds one of various FDA regulations.)*"*

"A common plan or conspiracy to seize the machinery of state, to commit crimes against the peace of the world, to blot a race out of existence, to enslave millions, and to subjugate and loot whole nations cannot be thought of in the same terms as the plotting of petty crimes, although the same underlying principles are applicable. The operation involves the manipulation of public opinion, the law of the state, the police power, industry, and finance. (Reminds one of various AMA activities and policies lasting decades.)*"*

"The defenders do not deny that these things happened, but it is contended that they 'just happened,' and that they were not the result of a common plan or conspiracy."

"Article 8 of the charter provides that the order of the government or of a superior shall not free a defendant from responsibility but can only be considered in mitigation."

"But it is urged that these defendants could not be in agreement on a common plan or in a conspiracy because they were fighting among themselves or belonged to different factions or cliques. Of course, it is not necessary that men should agree on everything in order to agree on enough things to make them liable for a criminal conspiracy. Unquestionably there were conspiracies within the conspiracy, and intrigues and rivalries and battles for power."

"The last stand of each defendant is that even if there was a conspiracy, he was not in it. It is therefore important in examining their attempts at avoidance of

responsibility to know, first of all, just what it is that a conspiracy charge comprehends and punishes."

"In conspiracy we do not punish one man for another man's crime. We seek to punish each for his own crime of joining a common criminal plan in which others also participated... the gist of the offense is participation in the formulation or execution of the plan. These are rules which every society has found necessary in order to reach men, like these defendants, who never get blood on their own hands but who lay plans that result in the shedding of blood."

"The list of defendants is made up of men who played indispensable and reciprocal parts in this tragedy."

"To escape the implications of their positions and the inference of guilt from their activities, the defendants are almost unanimous in one defense. The refrain is heard time and again: these men were without authority, without knowledge, without influence, indeed without importance."

"In the testimony of each defendant, at some point there was reached the familiar blank wall: nobody knew anything about what was going on. Time after time we have heard the chorus from the dock: 'I only heard about these things here for the first time.'"

"These men saw no evil, spoke none, and none was uttered in their presence."

"We have presented to this tribunal an affirmative case based on incriminating documents which are sufficient, if unexplained, to require a finding of guilt."

"They all speak with a Nazi double-talk with which to deceive the unwary. We must always look for hidden meanings.

"Besides outright false statements and double-talk, there are also other circumventions of truth in the nature of fantastic explanations and absurd profes-

sions."

"It is against such a background that these defendants now ask this tribunal to say that they are not guilty of planning, executing, or conspiring to commit this long list of crimes and wrongs. They stand before the record of this trial as bloodstained Gloucester stood by the body of his slain king. He begged of the widow, as they beg of you: 'Say I slew them not.' And the queen replied, 'Then say they were not slain. But dead they are.'"

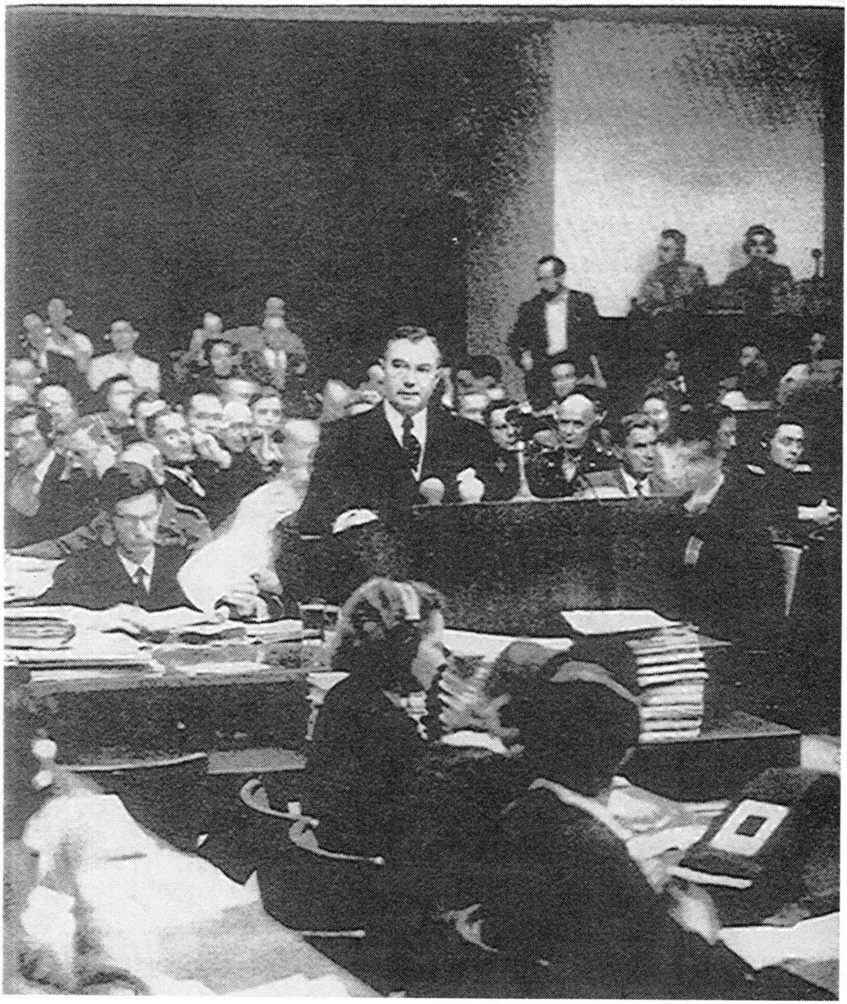

APPENDIX B: THE AMA's WAR AGAINST LIGHT THERAPY

In the 1920's, Dr. Kate Baldwin, the senior surgeon for 23 years at Philadelphia & Woman's Hospital — the oldest woman's hospital in America — introduced Light Therapy into the hospital. Its amazing results convinced her that Light Therapy was far superior to orthodox medical treatment. Unfortunately, the AMA was determined to suppress Light Therapy. In 1924 their attack was initiated in the *Journal of the AMA*.

In the next several years "medical politicians" went after the Light Therapy's creator and teacher of Dr. Baldwin, Dr. Baldwin herself, and all others who offered Light Therapy — which was, of course, just another form of "vibrational medicine" or "energy medicine." The "medical politicians," with the assistance of federal government agencies, succeeded in suppressing the new science and its threat to the Medical Monopoly. However, for decades to follow, millions of Americans suffered horribly as revolutionary, working treatments for burns, a long list of diseases, and every kind of human injury imaginable were denied them because the "medical politicians" at the AMA had chosen to put their own interests ahead of the public interest.

The following selected comments of Dr. Kate Baldwin, a half century before the revival of Light Therapy in the 1980's, should remind the reader of the magnitude of the crime perpetrated by the medical monopoly and its drug company and federal health agency co-conspirators in 20th century America.

> *"For centuries scientists have devoted untiring effort to discover means for the relief or cure of human ills and restoration of the normal functions. Yet in neglected*

light and color there is a potency far beyond that of drugs and serums. There are many shades of each color, and each is produced by a little different wave length. color waves may be tuned. Color is the simplest and most accurate therapeutic measure yet developed."

"After nearly thirty-seven years of active hospital practice and private practice in medicine and surgery, I can produce quicker and more accurate results with colors than with any or all other methods combined — and with less strain on the patient. The use of color in the treatment of burns — the burning sensation may be counteracted in from twenty to thirty minutes, and does not return. There is no question that light and color are important therapeutic media. Their adoption will be of advantage to the people." Paper written by Dr. Kate Baldwin and presented to the Medical Society of the State of Pennsylvania, October 12, 1926.

"I commenced to use Spectro-Chrome the latter part of 1920 or first of 1921 and it did not take me very long to decide that it was better than anything else I had. Any of the so-called Diseases, anything that is reasonably curable, it will cure and it will cure many things which Drugs and General Surgery and surgical work will not. In many cases of Cancer, Spectro-Chrome will cure it. I would close my office tonight never to see another sick person if I had to go back to old style Medicine and give up Spectro-Chrome." Testimony given by Kate Baldwin in 1931 at the trial of Dinshah P. Ghadiali, creator of the Light and Color Therapy system used by Dr. Baldwin.

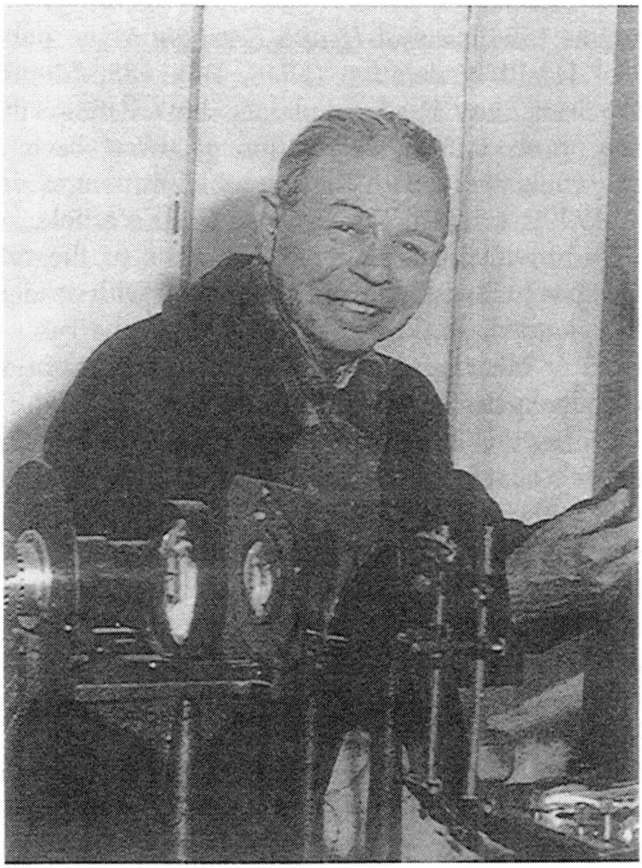

Happier Times

APPENDIX C: RIFE'S GREAT DISCOVERIES FROM A MODERN SCIENTIFIC PERSPECTIVE

In the August 1994 issue of Health Freedom News, published by the National Health Federation (NUF, Box 688, Monrovia, CA 91017), physicist Gary Wade explained how Rife's vibratory or coresonance or wave form destruction of dwarf bacteria in the 1930's also would work with the microbial structures defined by traditional, 1990's scientists as viruses. Wade's article, revised in 1996, clearly provided open-minded scientists of the future with powerful reasons to investigate and experiment with deadly diseases using Rife's approach to destroy them. Thus, real viruses linked to cancer, AIDS or other horrible, degenerative conditions were susceptible to an inexpensive, non-drug antidote.

Gary Wade has made a marvelous, unique contribution to the revival of Rife's suppressed scientific and medical breakthrough. In an Appendix to the article, which Mr. Wade encouraged and authorized people to "*copy and share*," he made a number of powerful statements which challenge traditional thinking and excuses by orthodox scientists that Rife's approach is nonsense and should be ignored or dismissed. Most of the technical details have been omitted from the selected quotations of Mr. Wade's Appendix offered here.

It is hoped that the common man or common woman reading Mr. Wade's words now, with the technical details relating to physics and microbes removed, will easily and quickly grasp how conventional scientists, doctors, and government health officials — abusing their authority — have played fast-and-loose with the public regarding Rife's historic discoveries and inventions. It is also hoped that those who read Mr. Wade's words now will quickly recognize how billions of dollars in research, clinical trials, and worthless, approved drugs by old boy networks within FDA and the National Institute of Health (NIH) have caused billions of dollars to be squandered on dangerous, immune-destroying drugs which didn't help the victims, but merely perpetuated a corrupt system.

Gary Wade asserted:

> *"The physical structure of virus capsids will show that they have construction which is particularly susceptible to destruction by structural resonant vibrations. Also a look at bacteria cell membrane and bacteria cell wall structure will suggest how and why bacteria are also susceptible to destruction by exposure to structural resonant vibrations."*
>
> *"When Rife exposed viruses to their most stressful mechanical oscillation mode, he could literally, while viewing them through his microscope, see them disintegrate and/or even explode."*
>
> *"To fully appreciate how and why a virus is so susceptible to its own mechanical structural resonant vibration frequency, it is necessary to apply some simple physics to the problem. All the physics that will be used is readily available in undergraduate physics mechanics text books, so I will simply state the results here."*
>
> *"With the proper choice of frequencies and relative intensity between frequencies and absolute intensities, we should be able to convert helical viruses into organic trash in one second or so."*
>
> *"HIV has three obvious periodic structures that can be attacked by structural resonant vibrations. It is practical to keep a person infected with a virus under continuous exposure to structural resonant vibrations for that virus. This can be achieved in several ways: 1)The person can wear a small inconspicuous ultrasound transducer unit, 2)Rife frequency instrument type 'light' can be installed at home or in the work place, and 3)Structural resonant vibration ultrasound can be carried by the room air. Now, if the virus is not allowed*

to infect new cells due to its destruction by structural resonant vibrations, then the body can potentially rid itself of the virus completely."

"Now on to bacteria destruction by structural resonant vibrations. From the remnants of Rife's work still publicly available, it is clear that Rife was able to destroy all bacteria he encountered using his frequency instrument. In other words, he could just as easily destroy viruses as bacteria with his frequency instrument. Someone or some institution will need to construct a modernized version of a Rife microscope and actually observe bacteria cell destruction by a Rife frequency instrument device to determine where the weak spots are in the bacteria cell wall which allow osmotic pressure to rupture the bacteria and spill its contents out."

"You should now understand how Rife, using his frequency instrument, was able by 1939 to destroy the viral and bacterial pathogens associated with 52 major diseases, including cancer."

"Rife's results were fully and completely verified by the 1934, 1935, and 1937 test clinical trials, which were carried out by the U.S.C. Medical School Special Medical Research Committee that oversaw the clinical trials."

"The responsibility for the deaths of, suffering by, and the financial ruin of tens upon tens of millions of people since 1937 clearly rests with the cowardly, greedy, and corrupt leadership/ownership of the medical industry. This includes pharmaceutical and insurance companies which have been major benefactors and pervaders of the greed and associated corruption."

"Rife treatments should be available everywhere right now! Now who do you think will resist Rife treatment implementation? Who do you think will attempt to and

has had laws, like the Weinberger law in California, passed so that you can only be treated for cancer by an allopathic medical doctor that only can use: 1) Surgery, 2) Radiation, and/or 3) Chemotherapy?"

* A comprehensive *Rife Technology Package* prepared by Gary Wade (for the technical minded) is available for $25 from:

Kursh Enterprises
801 Edie Drive
Duarte, CA 91010

APPENDIX D: HANSI

HANSI is a homeopathic developed by an Argentinean botanist Juan Hirshmann. Great numbers of people, including many with cancer, have benefited from its use. So stunning can be its results that American doctors with open minds have advocated its use and medical schools at quality American universities are conducting quiet "research."

Nevertheless, anti-alternative healing fanatics who have made careers out of attacking anything that is not conventional medicine already are denouncing HANSI. Who, again, gets the dirty deal? Patients throughout America who could have benefited from this potentially significant "energy healing" alternative but who simply were never given any information about it or the opportunity to have it in a modern hospital or clinic — that's who. The medical monopoly, protecting its own interests, not the patient's interest, imposed their power.

The following selected quotations will provide another glimpse into what is denied the American people.

From a presentation by Dewayne L. Hull, M.D. at Penn State University in October 1997:

> *"We are meeting to discuss treatment possibilities of a new paradigm for the coming millennium."*
>
> *"Financially speaking, the pharmaceutical and advertising industries have done quite well — while, over the past fifty years, the health of the people has deteriorated with the use of chemical pharmaceuticals."*
>
> *"If we are to develop a new treatment paradigm, we must sever the strings now being manipulated by the pharmaceutical industry — assisted by big government — and refocus our efforts on how one alters cellular*

one of these is called: HANSI, i.e. Homeopathic Activator of the Natural System Immune."

"HANSI is a multi-herbal produced in a homeopathic dilution. It has no side-effects and no toxicity."

"The effects of HANSI — with respect to solid cancers — are fascinating! That discussion is somewhat beyond the scope of this presentation. One would be almost unbelievably impressed when one observes those with the cellular diagnosis of cancer of the pancreas living without pain, maintaining their body weight and exhibiting extra energy. These people are living pretty much as you and I — and as much as five years after their diagnosis. It happens with regularity — when the patient avoids radical surgery, chemotherapy, and radiation and, instead, uses HANSI."

"I often contemplate what might be accomplished with a few of the billions of dollars we have spent on 'gene mapping.' One day, we could all see the light — visible or invisible to the human eye — because it all comes down to one fact — it's just a matter of resonance."

From "*HANSI: Argentina's Medical Miracle*," Townsend Letter for Doctors and Patients, October 1995:

"HANSI is the name Argentinean botanist Juan Hirshmann gave to his family of homeopathic treatments for a wide range of diseases, including cancer, AIDS, Chronic Fatigue Syndrome, arthritis, asthma, and hepatitis. In July of 1990, he opened his first clinic in Buenos Aires and began treating human cancer patients with HANSI".

"HANSI proved so effective that his first clinic was mobbed by cancer patients, alarming the government and requiring police for crowd control."

"HANSI International, Ltd., is a Bahamian company

with production and worldwide distribution rights to all of Juan Hirschmann's homeopathics. It imports its product (to America) under the FDA's personal use exemption rule."

From The Healing World of HANSI, a booklet published by the U.S. Information Office in Sarasota, Florida of HANSI International:

"What is HANSI? HANSI is a compound formed of the essences of plants and minerals found in the rain forests and deserts of Argentina, which are vastly diluted, energetically stored in water and introduced in tiny amounts into the human body. HANSI then activates, strengthens and balances the body's immune system, which becomes stimulated to perform its innate function —fighting disease and restoring homeostasis."

"HANSI has been clinically proven to be 100% not toxic and hence performs totally without harmful side effects."

"Research into alternative medicine has been neglected and discouraged in the United States, in favor of traditional medicine based upon chemical drugs. Fortunately that is not the case in other areas of the world."

"Since 1990, over 100,000 cancer patients have been treated in the Argentine clinics, with outstanding results and without any harmful side effects."

"Put at its simplest, HANSI normalizes/balances or modulates the immune system."

"HANSI cannot be synthesized (recreated chemically in a laboratory)."

"A French physician and scientist, Dr. Jacques Benveniste, confounded the world of immunology in 1995 with results of experiments."

"Allopathic or standard medicine effects relief from disease by introducing unnatural chemicals into the body to suppress disease organisms... Homeopathy induces the body to use its own defenses with tiny amounts of substances found in nature, and doing so entirely without unwanted side effects."

"Homeopathy is mainstream medicine in Germany, England, France and most other European countries."

"HANSI is an amalgam of many substances, and it can treat many different diseases, including the most difficult and serious ones."

"When Dr. Benveniste made his startling discovery that water can transfer and store molecular signals, he envisioned an imminent future when doctors would tap into the electromagnetic molecular communication system to perform surgery without knives, prevent disease without using vaccines, effect cures without drugs."

"He stated that his research could lead to 'the medicine of the future.'"

"HANSI is at least a bridge to that future, and more likely, is part of that future — now!"

APPENDIX E: CANCER SALVES: FUTURE ALTERNATIVE TO SURGERY?

Cancer Salves by Ingrid Naiman is a very careful explanation of the use of herbal salves for centuries in the treatment of cancer and especially as an alternative to surgery. By "drawing out" tumors, certain salves — when appropriately used and with the help of people experienced in the procedure — offer another valuable treatment in the emerging 21st century healing alternatives which 20th century conventional medicine has ignored because of medical politics and corrupt medical monopoly motives. It is hoped that Cancer Salves becomes the basis for serious scientific investigation of an exciting new mainstream therapy for people with cancer. Combined with energy medicine's revolutionary certainties, cancer salves may have a significant place among tomorrow's solidly scientific, foremost healing methods.

Cancer Salves is published by Seventh Ray Press, P. 0. Box 31007, Santa Fe, New Mexico 87594-1007, USA and distributed by North Atlantic Books, P.O. Box 12327, Berkeley, CA 94712. Web site addresses are: http://WWW.cancersalves.com and http://WWW.northatlanticbooks.com.

The following is from Cancer Salves:

> *"I personally do not believe that conventional medicine has extricated itself from the darker motivations of its predecessors: control of information with the objective of economic domination. Until it is able to clean its own house and police its own work, it will remain unreliable."*
>
> *"If the system were willing to question itself by critically assessing its reasons for failure, it would deserve*

the grants and monopolies it currently enjoys. However, studies suggest that its monopoly is a matter of money and politics rather than merit.

"In most cases, patients using the salves have never met another person who used the same approach; they do not know how to apply the salves or bandage the treatment sites; and they do not know how the salves work or what to expect. The present situation is, therefore, far from ideal for the patient; but hopefully this book will encourage more health care practitioners to develop expertise."

APPENDIX F: CHEMO-PATHOLOGY

In April 1999, the morons setting cancer policy issued a report stating that the greatest error in current scientific and medical treatment for cancer patients was???? (Three guesses for those who have read this book carefully.) Answer: The scientific experts decided that those with cancer were not getting enough chemotherapy and radiation after surgery.

USA Today newspaper reported on April 7, 1999, page 8D, in an article titled, "*Many Cancer Patients Miss Out On Best Care*" the following:

> *"Many of the more than 8 million people who will be treated for cancer this year won't get the therapies known to be most effective, says a major report."*
>
> *"Joseph Simone (is the) vice chairman of the National Cancer Policy Board. The board was created by the Institute of Medicine and the National Research Council, which advise the federal government on medical and scientific policy."*
>
> *"Simone says, 'It's common sense.'"*
>
> *"The report cites the underuse of therapies such as radiation and chemotherapy after surgery."*

The tragedy of permitting such ignorant, narrow-minded "experts" to control national policy and impose their flawed, biased beliefs on a nation remains the terrible reality of our times. The ongoing "medicide" continues its furious torture and killing of so many trusting cancer patients who are denied real choices and access to alternative cancer therapies which could cure their cancers forever.

Meanwhile, the Los Angeles Times' medical writer was misleading vast numbers of Southern California readers by headlining the same contrived chemo-pathology report as follows: "*Cancer Centers Rate Best.*" Still, pathetic as the journalism of medical writer Thomas H. Maugh II's was, at least it unwittingly revealed the forces behind the propaganda report: "*the Institute of Medicine report, commissioned by the National Cancer Institute, the American Cancer Society, the Centers for Disease Control and Prevention, and two pharmaceutical companies.*" Los Angeles Times, (April 12, 1999), p. S2.

The following week, it was announced that the cancer elite's love for bone-marrow transplants for breast cancer had proven to be an essentially worthless, painful and super expensive ($100,000) failure. The results of clinical trials revealed:

> "*No significant overall increase in survival. The transplants are not themselves an anticancer therapy. Rather, they support the patient's body, allowing doctors to treat tumors much more aggressively. In such cases, physicians use as much as twenty times the normal dose of cancer drugs.*" Los Angeles Times, (April 16, 1999), pp. Al, All.

Chemo-Pathology combined with self-serving surgeon fanaticism! Bone marrow transplants were actually nothing but medical madness masquerading as very, very lucrative (for the doctors) "scientific" experimentation.

APPENDIX G: DRUG MEDICINE A LEADING CAUSE OF DEATH

It appeared in the *Journal of the AMA* for April 15, 1998. It was an article which examined the number of deaths in America caused by a reaction to drug medicine. The article was based on research combining 32 years (!) and 39 studies of what is termed "*Adverse drug reactions*" (ADR) in hospital patients which killed them. The conclusion was that drug medicine might be the 4th leading cause of death after heart disease, cancer and stroke.

It was fitting that the AMA published such a stunning, horrible statistic. After all, the AMA had played a huge role in suppressing many truly wonderful healing therapies in order that the AMA and its members could benefit from drug therapy. Now the chickens were coming home to roost (and roast). The American people were wising up to the failures of orthodox drug medicine and seeking alternatives. The crimes of doctors, scientists and government health officials, in forcing drug medicine on the American people for so many decades, was gradually becoming known.

Here is a sample from the April 15, 1998 *JAMA* article which hits the medical monopolists like a hammer:

> *"Adverse drug reactions (ADA) may be a major cause of death in hospitalized patients. We have found that serious ADR's are frequent and more so than generally recognized. Fatal ADR's appear to be between the fourth and sixth leading cause of death. Their incidence has remained stable over the last 30 years."*

Meanwhile, as the awful facts and truth of what the medical monopoly and its drug obsession had done to millions of Americans over decades and decades began to become hardened statistical data, those still dominating conventional cancer therapy and research refused to concede an inch. Incredibly, they organized to bleed the American people of more money for their worthless, blinders-on cancer priorities.

The Seattle Times, on October 15, 1998, published an article originating at The Washington Post. According to the article, "*165 experts, including some of the nation's top researchers*" had collectively written a report. The report recommended the budget at the National Cancer Institute be increased from its yearly $2.5 billion for "*research*" to $10 billion by the year 2003. All this while therapies which actually cured cancer were ignored, suppressed and described in media press releases with overt, consciously contrived lies and disinformation.

The brainwashed, uninformed, high paid television doctors hawked the big lie of drug medicine to countless vulnerable Americans. It was a tragedy rivaling the Inquisition's mindless murder of millions in Europe during the Middle Ages. Here is a sample of what television doctors casually prescribe — Dr. Robert Arnot, the "*trusted CBS News Medical correspondent*" blathering the standard propaganda. Dr. Arnot baldly encourages cancer patients to take conventional treatment first and then, if that doesn't work, to enroll in the National Cancer Institute's experimental trials. The quotation is from his silly book The Best Medicine, pages 266, 268, 270.

> *"Make sure you receive the maximum benefit from conventional therapies first. The National Cancer Institute believes that thousands of patients die each year because their doses of chemotherapy were inadequate. This is the single biggest mistake in chemotherapy. Patients can find the best experimental therapies at America's most prestigious cancer institutes. You may be one of the first to benefit from a powerful new treatment."*

So the “medicide” continues and the people who have been miraculously cured of cancer by alternative therapies are studiously ignored by the medical fundamentalists, their scientific cohorts, and the government bureaucrats controlling the money and regulating what therapies are permitted and what therapies are forbidden.

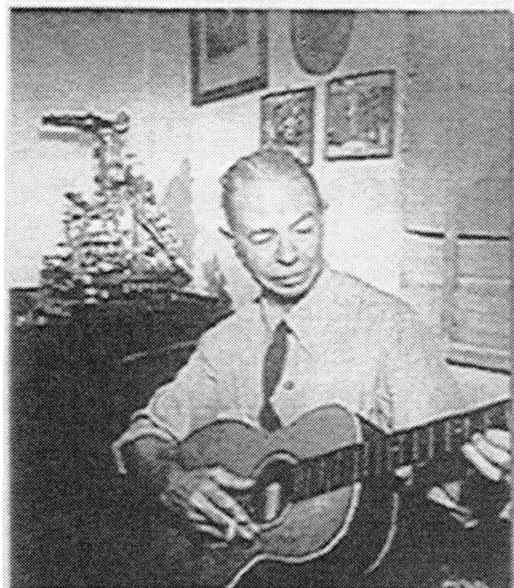

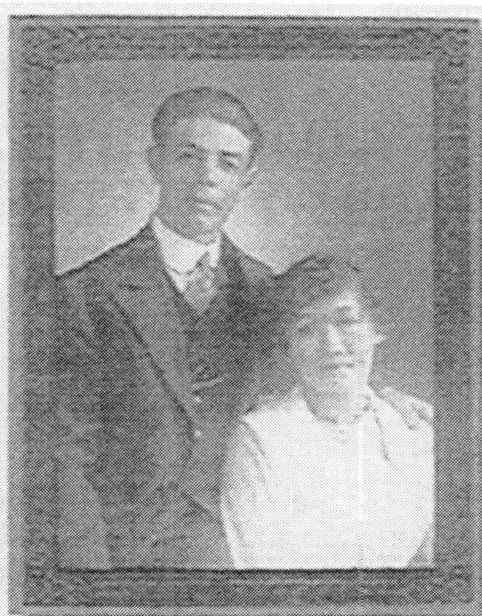

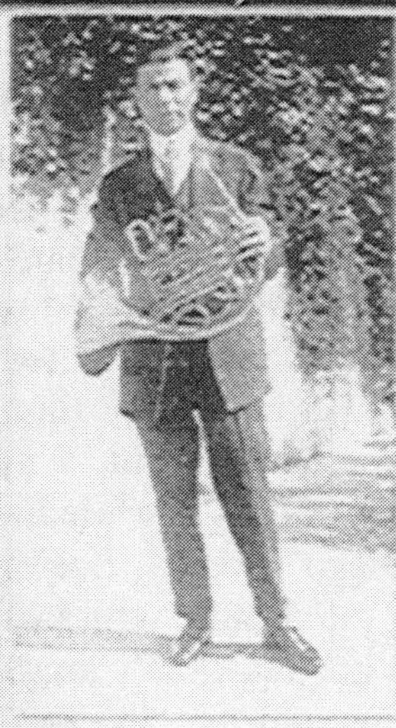

Royal Raymond Rife

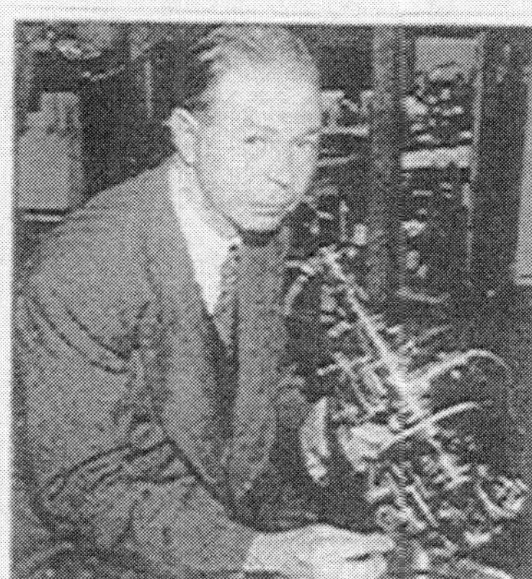

APPENDIX H:
WHAT MIGHT HAVE BEEN — RIFE ARRIVES ON THE NATIONAL SCENE

In the Spring of 1931, the nationally distributed magazine Popular Science broke the story of Royal R. Rife's scientific genius and the medical miracles which his work, discoveries and inventions made possible. Soon after, a number of prominent scientists began their journeys to San Diego in order to see for themselves what Rife had accomplished and what the future promised.

Everything that happened in the remainder of the decade of the 1930's relating to Rife originated with that stunning article in Popular Science — the development of the team which comprised the University of Southern California's Special Medical Research Committee; the cancer clinics which validated Rife's Energy Medicine cure as the mysterious microbe responsible for many, if not all, cancers was painlessly destroyed and people diagnosed with terminal cancer were completely healed of their cancers; the verification of the Rife microscope's power and national publication in Science magazine of that fact by one of the Mayo Clinic's most eminent scientists; the organized suppression of Energy Medicine by the A.M.A., culminating in the San Diego Medical Society's invasion of doctor's offices and threatening the doctors with loss of their medical licenses and jail terms if the doctors didn't immediately cease using Rife's powerful healing instrument; and finally, the 1939 trial which destroyed Rife and halted his medical and scientific discoveries from being widely distributed and integrated into mainstream medicine throughout America for decades and decades to come — it all flowed from the one breakthrough article in Popular Science in the Spring of 1931.

Here is an edited selection from that June 1931 issue of Popular Science with its absolutely stunning scientific announcement of what the, until then, unknown genius Royal R. Rife was doing:

> *"On a six-by-eight foot screen in a darkened room appeared a spherical object. It resembled a gray, indoor baseball, crisscrossed in all directions by fine threads of silk. Slowly and aimlessly it rotated."*
>
> *"'The spore of the bacterium that causes lockjaw,' came a voice from the loudspeaker of the motion picture apparatus. 'Watch it!'"*
>
> *"A dozen physicians and laboratory workers leaned forward. The sphere swelled. When it had become six inches or more in diameter on the screen, a dark line appeared across its middle. It parted. From it emerged a dark bar, nearly as long as the diameter of the sphere, spinning on its long axis — the cylinder-shaped germ of tetanus, or lockjaw. For what was probably the first time, a movie had shown the lockjaw spore hatching."*
>
> *"We were in the laboratory of R. R. Rife at San Diego, California. He is a pioneer in the art of making motion pictures of the microscopically small. Rife began building his own microscopes in a laboratory fitted up in a room over the garage. In this little room, he has today more than $50,000 worth of microscopes and cameras. Most of them he built himself."*
>
> *"For ten years he has worked to capture in motion pictures what the eye sees through the most powerful microscopes. He has succeeded and his work has won the recognition from the medical profession. Now doctors may sit at ease in comfortable chairs and watch bacteria in their native surroundings on a motion picture screen. There they may compare their own observations of disease germs taken from patients with the life history of these microbes preserved on motion picture film. It is estimated that the time required to diagnose certain diseases may be cut from days to*

hours by the use of the films."

"Whence came the actors in these strange movies? Rife propagates and rears all the microbes he studies in an incubating plant of his own design. Deadly germs housed in jars are nursed as carefully as the frailest child. Delicate thermostats control the warmth of ovens in which the germs are kept active, or the coolness of refrigerators in which they lie dormant. 'If the electric current holds out,' Rife told me, 'These microorganisms will be alive a million years from today, without the interference of a human hand.'"

"When he is ready to make a movie, Rife places a small colony of disease germs on a quartz slide. Then he picks up one or more with a human hair, the tiniest obtainable, which is split lengthwise and mounted in a chuck beneath the lens of his microscope. Slowly he lowers the strange pair of tweezers onto the slide. Its halves part. Between them one or a few microbes lodge. Lifting out the hair, Rife transfers them to the stage of the micro-movie camera, and he is ready to film the life history of a germ."

"An electric light of 2,000 candlepower falls upon the center of this microscopic movie studio — a tiny spot on the thin slab of transparent quartz that bears the germs. Above it, sixteen of the finest quartz lenses obtainable, immersed in glycerin, magnify the dimensions of each germ 12,000 times. Designed by Rife himself, this apparatus is one of the most powerful microscopes in the world; its magnification compares with the 2,000-diameter enlargement of microscopes commonly used in research laboratories and in medical examinations."

"Either as he makes the film or afterward, Rife records a lecture to accompany it upon a sound strip synchronized with the picture."

"He showed me a quartz slide bearing several hundred typhus germs."

"'We have weighed them on extremely delicate balances,' Rife added. 'The weight of these disease germs averages one-184-trillionth part of an ounce.'"

"How various rays affect the lives and activities of disease germs was another thing that Rife wanted to find out."

"While the X-rays had no effect on lockjaw germs, and ultraviolet or invisible light rays merely halted their development, Rife discovered that the green ray would destroy the microbes. Now he is making a movie of that operation."

"Rife has devised a magnetic compass so delicate that it can be used to study the electricity and magnetism in living germs. He suggests that if the electrical make-up of certain dangerous germs is learned, it may someday be possible to destroy them in the human body by applying small doses of electricity."

As time would prove, that last paragraph in the Popular Science article was prophetic. Rife did learn how to electromagnetically destroy the microbes which caused the diseases responsible for some of humanity's greatest suffering. But the Medical Monopoly didn't want it. So they destroyed Rife, suppressed his breakthrough science and inflicted untold agony on millions of Americans as well as people throughout the world until the late 1980's and 1990's, when the revival of Rife's awesome, historic discoveries exploded anew. Now, as the 21st century begins, this promises to be a significant feature in a new medicine and new approach to providing millions with a level of health never previously known by the majority of human beings. Hurrah for Rife. Those of us now living and generations unborn owe him our everlasting gratitude.

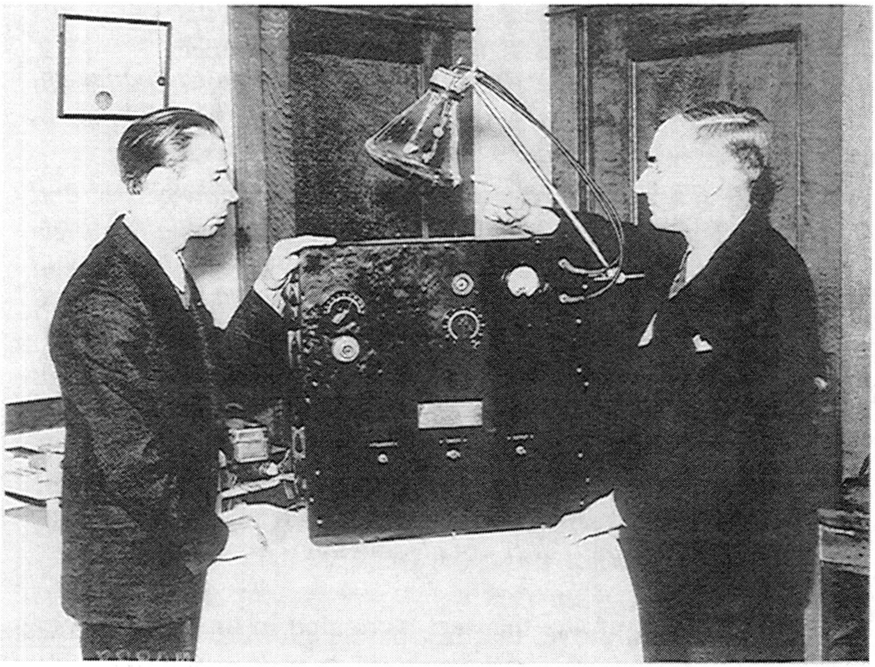

APPENDIX I: MAINSTREAM NEWSPAPER BEGINS "SNIFFING" THE RIFE PHENOMENON IN 1997

Sixty-six years after Popular Science gave the American nation and its people the incredible news of what Royal R. Rife had already done in 1931, a modern, mainstream newspaper began "*sniffing*" that something "*newsworthy*" and worth reporting was occurring in the grassroots alternative health movement relating to "*someone*" named Royal R. Rife who lived decades ago. That breakthrough story at last ended the Medical Monopoly's censorship.

Nevertheless, the breakout story on Royal R. Rife which occurred in 1997 was very, very cautious and filled with excuses concerning why medical "*professionals*" would be reluctant to investigate Rife, even if his long-lost therapy could cure cancer. Tragically, the article — while a breakthrough — did demonstrate the media's conspicuous role in silently permitting the medical crime of the century. Thus, the crack in the modern media wall regarding Rife was instructive.

The following few selected quotes are from this article which appeared in the Sunday magazine section ("*Tropic*") of the Miami Herald on August 10, 1997. The readers of this book, now aware of all the corruption and terrible mayhem perpetrated by medical interests for so long, should benefit from seeing how facts describing Rife's revival are handled so superficially even today, with a kind of agonized, groveling, shameful inclusion of the official medical political line. Sadly, the true story of Rife probably remains a long way from being told in the American press unless some courageous reporters, editors and publisher of a major, mainstream newspaper choose to be courageous and dare to change the world forever by telling the truth of Rife's genius, suppression and now revitalized science exploding on the Internet and in countries around

"Dr. Steven N. Rosenberg, a Board Certified obstetrician/gynecologist and a past president of the Fort Lauderdale OB/GYN Society has been observing Ratelle and the machine for the past four months."

"'The word 'cure' means seeing results over a long period of time,' he says. 'We haven't seen the long-term results yet. But I have seen it eliminate the presence of cancer.'"

"What is this mysterious machine?"

"The Rife machine — also known as the Rife Frequency Generator, the Rife Beam Ray or the Rife Resonator — is based on a prototype invented by a scientist named Dr. Royal Raymond Rife in San Diego in the 1930's."

"According to Rife, who died in 1971, his machine can kill a bacterium or virus by generating the appropriate electrical frequency — the pathogen's 'Mortal Oscillatory Rate' — and destroying it through resonance."

"Dr. Rife said in a May 11, 1938, article in the San Diego Evening Tribune, 'We can say that these frequencies have been shown to possess the power of killing disease organisms when tuned to an exact wavelength.'"

"Rife based this claim, in part, on a 1934 clinical study under the auspices of a 'Special Medical Research Committee' at the University of Southern California."

"No such committee currently exists at the USC, and a reference librarian at the USC Medical School could not locate any mention of Royal Rife."

"In a 1987 book about Rife, The Cancer Cure That Worked: Fifty Years of Suppression, author Barry Lynes claims that the records of Rife's clinical studies 'mysteriously disappeared' from the university in the 1940's, one part of what he portrays as a massive conspiracy against Rife by the medical establishment."

"Since the 1930's, there have been no significant

professional papers published about the Rife machine and no significant controlled studies of it."

"Little of Rife's own work remains for posterity. His discovery went virtually unnoticed for more than fifty years, until 1987, when Lynes' book about Rife and his machine was published."

"So why is the Rife machine still a mystery in the medical establishment? Dr. S. A. Williams, 77, a retired family practice MD in West Palm Beach, said it's simply because nobody has taken the time to study it."

"'They don't bother to read about it — they call it hocus pocus,' said Williams. 'And they're making good money. Why do they have to bother with anything else?'"

"Jim Benson, former FDA deputy commissioner, said the FDA is not trying to keep legitimate devices out of the public hands. 'But it's possible they would have a tough time getting a clinical study going.'"

"Dr. Rosenberg, who plans to study the Rife machine further, also does not believe there is a government conspiracy against the Rife machine, just a reluctance to accept anything out of bounds of conventional medicine."

"'People get comfortable with what they're used to,' says Rosenberg, 'It's not so much a conspiracy as it is the natural difficulty in changing patterns of belief.'"

"In a 1994 report, the American Cancer Society 'strongly urges individuals with cancer not to seek treatment with such devices.'"

"Ratelle knew that by cooperating for this story, breaking nine years of silence, he risked drawing some unwanted attention from the FDA and/or AMA."

"He says he is dedicated to his clients. He has seen around 1,250 clients in his nine years operating the Rife machine."

The sad part of this story is that the reporter or editor could have verified so much more concerning Rife. But it was easier to be superficial regarding Rife's discoveries, inventions and genius. To be forthright and honest would have stirred a hornet's nest from the medical interests and those 165 "*top cancer researchers*" who were seeking to get the annual cancer "*research*" budget of the National Cancer Institute up to $10 billion a year. So the *Miami Herald* focused on one courageous underground Rife proponent who — for nine years, with no funds, no hard core research, no microscope, no lab work doing blood analysis, etc., etc., etc. — did what his heart and soul knew was right. America was built by such people — citizens who were free and not intimidated by criminal interests.

The Lancet, one of the world's foremost medical journals, published the following observation in its March 6, 1993 issue:

> *"The professionalisation of orthodox medicine and the concurrent marginalisation of its alternatives has had more to do with institutional power than with the merits of what was available. The course of alternative medicine can only be understood through study of the history of medical institutions and the politics of vested interests."*

So true. So sadly true.

But the times are a-changing. And tomorrow's healing therapies will be different and will reflect the patient's interest and rights, not the Medical Monopoly's interest, greed and tyrannical violation of people's bodies.

Now, if only one or more mainstream newspaper would dare to publish the real Rife story and the real truths concerning other therapies which cure cancer. The world would change overnight.

Thank God the Internet is doing what mainstream newspapers and television are afraid to do.

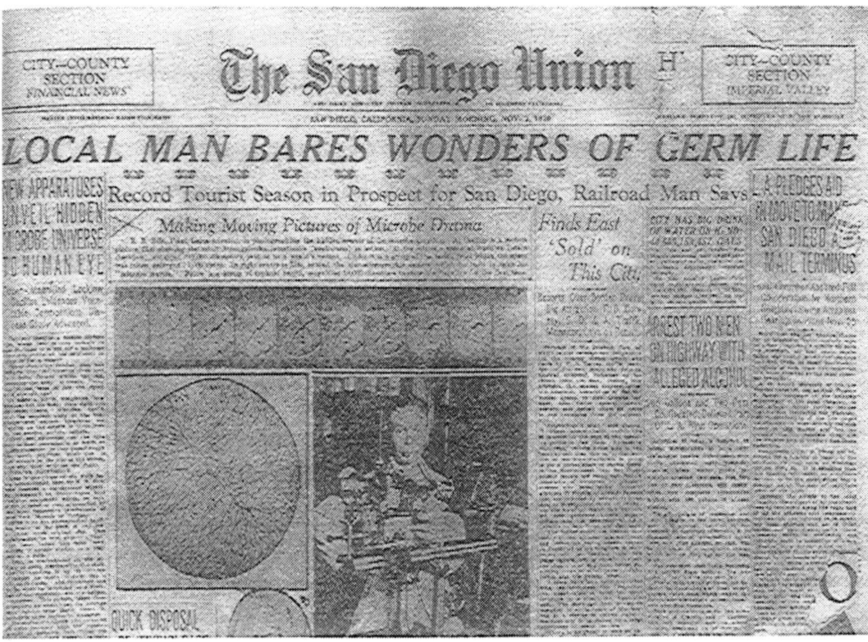

CITY—COUNTY SECTION FINANCIAL NEWS

The San Diego Union

CITY—COUNTY SECTION IMPERIAL VALLEY

LOCAL MAN BARES WONDERS OF GERM LIFE

NEW APPARATUSES UNVEIL HIDDEN MICROBE UNIVERSE TO HUMAN EYE

Record Tourist Season in Prospect for San Diego, Railroad Man Says

Making Moving Pictures of Microbe Drama

Finds East 'Sold' on This City

L.A. PLEDGES AID IN MOVE TO MAKE SAN DIEGO A MAIL TERMINUS

ARREST TWO MEN ON HIGHWAY WITH ALLEGED ALCOHOL

QUICK DISPOSAL

APPENDIX J:
Nanobacteria — RIFE VINDICATION

In October 1998, the Ottawa Sun continued the media's more than half century record of putting forth distortions and lies as it demonstrated cowardly obedience to the cancer establishment whenever the subject was Royal R. Rife. As the 2nd International Rife Conference gathered more than 200 people from around the world — including a large percentage who were either physicians or people with advanced degrees — into British Columbia, the newspaper of Canada's capital shamed the basic journalistic standards by emphasizing in their coverage the know-nothing remarks of a spokeswoman for the Canadian Cancer Society. "*The equipment isn't even worthy of research dollars, a society spokeswoman says*," reported the Ottawa Sun on October 16, 1998.

That public relations propaganda line echoed the misleading statements of a cancer "*expert*" and former president of the American Cancer Society who was featured in an American television show on Rife in 1997. Strange Universe was the first nationally syndicated television program which broadcast original black-and-white film footage of Rife in his 1930's laboratory. But the scared producers had to balance the Rife breakout by including the American Cancer Society's ex-president who denounced Rife and instead encouraged those with cancer to take the establishment medicine's "*experimental*" chemotherapy. It was a pathetic demonstration of intellectual dishonesty and ignorance masquerading as expertise.

Unfortunately, both the Canadian and American Cancer Society propagandists were not keeping up with modern science. While their organizations collected tens of millions and hundreds of millions of dollars every year from trusting citizens of the two neighboring nations, and then wasted the money on bloated administrative salaries, real estate speculation, and safe, non-threatening cancer research, real scientists on the cutting edge of hard science were discovering that Rife might have been right all along. Oh-oh, perhaps the Canadian and American Cancer Society spokespersons would have to plead, "*I didn't know*" sometime in the future. A refrain from Nuremberg.

Of course the pathetic, poor journalism of the Ottawa Sun and countless other major newspapers could not be excused. Millions of lives were lost while the newspapers parroted disinformation from the cancer establishment. Nevertheless, the hurricane-force vindication of Rife was continuing to build.

In April 1999, the Los Angeles Times reported that top researchers in America and in other countries were studying "*Nanobacteria.*" Nanobacteria sure sounded suspiciously like what Rife was attacking in the 1930's and saving people's lives left and right — until the medical associations decided "*electronic healing*" or "*energy medicine*" wasn't good for their organizations' wallets and bank accounts.

On April 22, 1999, the Los Angeles Times reported that the Nanobacteria "*are extremely small, some as small as a virus.*"

Of course the cost of a belated recognition of Rife could not even be measured — millions of dead and decades of agony. The "*new*" and "*hot*" research area of Nanobacteria, acknowledged by the Los Angeles Times in the spring of 1999, was exactly where Rife's brilliant eye, staring through his magnificent microscope, had been focused — in the 1920's and the 1930's!

In order for the reader to grasp the incredible arrogance and stupidity of the American and Canadian Cancer Society officials, and their pitiless contempt for cancer patients in stating Rife was worthless and not deserving of even "*research dollars,*" let us look at tuberculosis in the 1999 context of Rife and Nanobacteria.

Tuberculosis has existed since ancient times. It has been found in the remains of mummies from the Egyptian dynasties and was described by Hippocrates, the father of medicine, in Greece hundreds of years before Christ's birth.

Then, after all these centuries of suffering, in 1882 the German doctor Robert Koch discovered its cause — a bacteria. Koch became famous overnight.

In 1890, Koch announced he had a TB serum which would cure the disease. But, unfortunately, he was wrong; for some reason which he could not understand, his serum did not work. People and animals died.

Tuberculosis was the leading cause of death in America during the first decade of the 20th century. Gradually however, with drug therapy and better living conditions, TB was controlled. That is, until the late 1980's, when drug-resistant forms of TB, weakened human immune systems, and urban crowding resulted in a resurgence of tuberculosis.

In the 1990's, approximately 3 million human beings around the globe still died of tuberculosis every year. Several more millions became infected every year and yet, hard as it may be to believe, it is possible that TB could be totally eradicated just as was smallpox. Why? How? Because Rife had discovered something which Koch in the 1880's and 1890's did not know and certainly could not prove.

Royal R. Rife's super microscope enabled him to study the TB bacteria without staining (and killing) it with chemical dyes. Rife observed the TB bacteria in its live state and — because his microscope had such great magnification and resolution — he observed a tiny, virus-sized microbe escape from the bacteria when the bacteria died. Rife learned how to devitalize or destroy both the bacteria which caused TB and the deadly smaller form (Nanobacteria or dwarf bacteria) which escaped when Robert Koch or others attacked only the large bacteria associated with TB.

How did Royal R. Rife kill these two microbes at the same time? He used specific frequencies which were deadly to both the large bacteria and its smaller, dwarf form without harming anything else in the body.

Surely it is time to take a new look with objective, scientific eyes at what Royal R. Rife offered the world in the 1930's! The three million people who will die this year of TB, while the establishment medicine propagandists monopolize the media, at least deserve some unbiased, factual investigation. A fair investigation of what

Rife offered the world decades and decades ago will indicate he cured TB for the first time in the history of the world.

Millions of human lives have been lost because of medical myopia and medical politics.

Here are Rife's own words describing the cure for TB which is available for the world today simply by resurrecting his work:

> *"I worked a great deal on tuberculosis. I isolated the poison molecule. Koch originally produced the vaccines and anti-toxins that would kill the bacilli of tuberculosis, but they would also kill the patient. Simply because with any known method or means that you release from tuberculosis the so-called poisons, they react upon the dead bodies of the rod form and produce toxemia and death. I finally found an electronic frequency that would kill these bacteria. If two of the frequencies are used simultaneously, or one right after (the other), over the same carrier wave, the patient gets well. If you use either frequency individually you either kill the patient or you accomplish nothing."*

In 1934, Florence Seibert purified Koch's 1890 serum. This became the basis for the modern TB skin test which determines whether a person currently has or ever was infected by the tuberculosis bacteria. X-rays and other diagnostic tools then can determine if the person has an active infection. A complicated drug treatment is then initiated which lasts for months. Obviously the poor, the homeless, the drug addicted — those in America most prone to tuberculosis — or the many millions crowded together in poor, undeveloped countries — are not likely to be able to afford or be psychologically inclined to follow such a doctor-dependent regimen.

So TB grows and grows and drug-resistant forms of TB threaten the world with a new "White Plague."

But Rife's method for curing TB could be an easy, worldwide procedure which, in time, could end the "White Plague" of tuberculosis forever — after all these centuries.

In the early 1990's Florence Seibert was inaugurated into the Woman's Hall of Fame in Seneca, N.Y. for her lifetime scientific achievements. A few years prior to this honor, she made the following public statement regarding Royal R. Rife:

> *"I had no knowledge of the Rife microscope until a short time ago, and I have been around in the scientific world! I'm so glad it is not lost. I encourage all to do what they can to support this research."*

It is time to eradicate tuberculosis from our planet forever. We have that opportunity now by resurrecting and reclaiming Rife's great discovery. Scientists and physicians around the world should lead this long overdue initiative but the people of the world, those suffering from TB as well as those fortunate enough to be spared, should be active in this struggle also.

The official silence of mainstream medicine regarding Rife and his TB cure has lasted for too many decades.

The admission by the mainstream media that Nanobacteria is a hot, new research subject in universities around the world should help vindicate Rife, regardless of what the dunces at the Canadian and American Cancer Societies say to keep the public misinformed.

> Oh, and by the way, law enforcement officials and "health" officials in California have jailed Asian refugees for up to 10 months for refusing to take expensive TB drug medicine. "*Treatment for the milder form of TB can take up to nine months and cost $60,000, health officials said. For the drug-resistant form, treatment can last up to 36 months, cost more than $200,000 and cause nausea and other side effects.*" Los Angeles Times, (May 31, 1999), pp. A3, A24.
>
> This outrage and abuse of Constitutional rights — jailing people without a trial based on a health official's administrative order — is the result of the California Medical

Association (CMA), allied with drug companies and state government flunkies, sponsoring mayhem in order to keep Rife's miraculous wave-form therapies from California citizens and American citizens — all at California taxpayer's expense!

Meanwhile, the National Institutes of Health, with a yearly budget of $15.6 billion (*L.A. Times*, June 4, 1999) keep the $$ flowing to its "chemo-nut" "researchers."

"Yuck, yuck," they chuckle, as they continue to steal Americans' tax dollars for a classic, gigantic swindle. $200,000 per patient!!!!

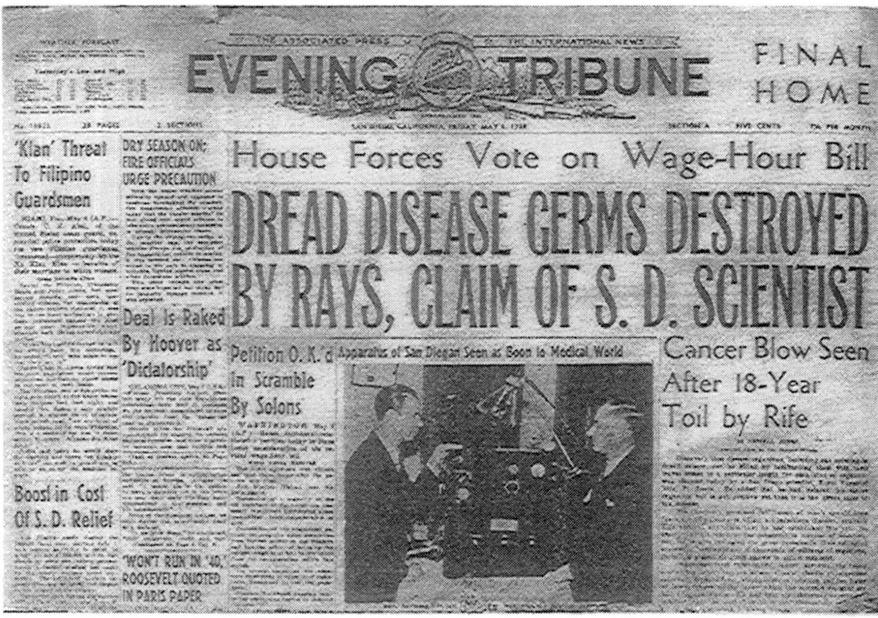

THE ASSOCIATED PRESS — THE INTERNATIONAL NEWS

EVENING TRIBUNE

FINAL HOME

House Forces Vote on Wage-Hour Bill

DREAD DISEASE GERMS DESTROYED BY RAYS, CLAIM OF S. D. SCIENTIST

'Klan' Threat To Filipino Guardsmen

DRY SEASON ON; FIRE OFFICIALS URGE PRECAUTION

Deal Is Raked By Hoover as 'Dictatorship'

Petition O.K.'d In Scramble By Solons

Apparatus of San Diegan Seen as Boon to Medical World

Cancer Blow Seen After 18-Year Toil by Rife

Boost in Cost Of S. D. Relief

'WON'T RUN IN '40,' ROOSEVELT QUOTED IN PARIS PAPER

APPENDIX K: THE RIFE RAY

On May 6, 1938, the San Diego Evening Tribune told its readers what newspapers in America and Canada were still afraid to publish in 1999!

On the front page, with large headlines and a picture, the newspaper informed its readers of Rife's historic work. One honest reporter had been monitoring and communicating with Rife since the first clinical trial in 1934. That trial — utilizing Rife's Ray on people with cancer — had resulted in 16 of 16 cancer patients being cured. Every single one of those 16 cancer patients had been diagnosed as "terminal" by orthodox medicine.

Here's an excerpt from that historic article in 1938 which described how Rife's precisely tuned ray destroyed specific microbes responsible for specific diseases, including cancer:

> *"Rife thinks that the lethal frequencies for various disease organisms are, as in the sound waves, coordinates of frequencies existing in the organisms themselves, when the ray is directed upon them, they are seen to behave very curiously; some kinds do literally disintegrate, and others writhe as if in agony and finally gather together in deathly unmoving clusters.*
>
> *"Brief exposure to the tuned frequencies, Rife commented, brings the fatal reactions. In some organisms, it happens in seconds.*
>
> *"After the organisms have been bombarded, the laboratory reports show, they are dead. They have become devitalized — no longer exhibit life, do not propagate their kind and produce no disease when introduced into the bodies of experimental animals.*
>
> *"Now, he reported, the mortal oscillatory rates for many, many organisms have been found and recorded*

> *and the ray can be tuned to a germ's recorded frequency and turned upon that organism with the assurance that the organism will be killed."*

Yet, sadly, 60 years later, the National Cancer Institute (NCI) continued to ignore Rife and worked diligently to induce cancer patients into experimental chemotherapy trials which would kill most of them.

During Congressional hearings in 1998 on this continuing atrocity perpetrated by NCI "experts" whose high salaries were paid by American taxpayers, Ralph Moss exposed the dirty little secret which the NCI desk murderers didn't want the American public ever to learn.

Here are some terrible truths provided by Ralph Moss in testimony before the House Committee on Government Reform and Oversight.

> *"If you read the statements of the NCI, they urgently appeal to cancer patients to join their clinical trials. In fact, there is little chance of therapeutic benefit to patients in such trials. Studies in both the United States and Japan have shown that only about one percent of patients in Phase I clinical trials have a complete response to the treatment, and only about five percent have any response at all."*
>
> *"I want to call your attention to the fact that these trials can be very dangerous for patients. The drugs approved by the FDA for treating cancer are all toxic. This is the 'scientific' approach of NCI. Not surprisingly, there is tremendous resistance among patients and doctors to such trials. Only three to five percent of cancer patients go into them.*
>
> *"No wonder cancer patients today are desperately looking for alternatives."*
>
> *"You can be sure that one of the reasons the NCI and FDA so hate these alternative treatments is that they*

> *siphon away "adventurous" patients who might otherwise go into clinical trials."*
>
> *"Historically, all of the agencies involved in the war on cancer have lied about the nature of these alternatives. Tests were only performed under duress (often because the Congress insisted) and these tests were at best ill-conceived and at worst marked by outright fraud."*
>
> *"The NCI along with its police partner, the FDA, is the great roadblock to the examination of promising new ways of treating cancer."*

In 1999, 178,000 American women will learn they have invasive breast cancer. More than 43,500 will die. Yet the breast cancer organizations which raise money, march in huge parades, have big beauty product corporate sponsors, and numerous Hollywood celebrities pitching for them, continue to finance traditional drug "researchers." Letters sent to their highest officials concerning Rife are not answered. The same goes for the "superstars" of the government health agencies.

In 1992, Dr. Jane Henney was informed of the significant discoveries in the 1930s of Royal R. Rife and how his original approach to curing cancer deserved a new evaluation.

Dr. Jane Henney was a cancer specialist, having worked for almost ten years at the National Cancer Institute and eventually becoming its Deputy Director. She had just joined FDA in 1992 when she was informed of Royal R. Rife's work in the 1930's.

Dr. Jane Henney replied politely in a written communication concerning Royal R. Rife and his incredible discovery, but she showed no interest in pursuing his work or encouraging others even to investigate it. Despite 10,000 Americans dying of cancer that week and the next week and the week after, week after week, year after year, Rife's discoveries didn't stir the slightest curiosity on her part.

Dr. Jane Henney worked for FDA from 1992 to 1994 as one of the

Commissioner's closest deputies. In 1994 she left the FDA and took a new position at the University of New Mexico where she consolidated its various hospitals. Cancer remained one of her areas of focus.

In June 1998, Dr. Jane Henney was appointed the Commissioner of the FDA.

In those 6 years from 1992 to 1998, 3 million Americans had died of cancer, billions of dollars had been spent on cancer "research," and not one penny had gone to Rife-related investigation of what Rife had discovered and proved in the 1930's. (On January 24, 1999, the Los Angeles Times reported "*More than $16 billion is available for medical research*" from the U. S. government.)

It may soon be time for democratic institutions in America to begin considering the dismaying truth that the name of the game for many medical specialists and government health officials is, and has been, power and privilege, not the interests of people who have some terrible ailments and diseases. It is a frightening evaluation which needs to be honestly undertaken very soon.

> *"The culture of clinical trials is plagued by conflicts of interest. Drug companies pay doctors handsomely — sometimes as much as $6,000 per patient — to test new drugs."* "*Dying for a cure*," U.S. News & World Report, (October 11, 1999), p. 36.

APPENDIX L: TOXIC FOLLIES: THE BREAST CANCER TORTURE SCHEMES

In Appendix F (Chemo-Pathology), it was mentioned that the years and years of experimenting on women with breast cancer using bone marrow transplant as an excuse for high dose chemotherapy had finally been shown to be a failure. While many doctors and scientists had known for years and years that it was nothing but another financially lucrative breast cancer torture scheme, most had chosen to stay silent.

The media also were guilty of keeping its publishing and broadcasting channels tightly closed. Why upset the medical powers by telling the public the truth? Why inform desperate women with breast cancer that they were being lied to, and misled into torturous, unnecessary, useless treatment?

But, the media knew the facts. They simply chose to sit on the sidelines and not raise a stink while cruel, inhuman procedures were passed off as "experimental" at a nominal fee of $50,000 to $150,000 per experiment.

Here is Newsweek, the national weekly magazine, in 1990 (!), clearly revealing that they had a comprehensive grasp of the reality:

> *"Doctors remove some of the patient's bone marrow, then administer extremely high doses of chemotherapy. ABMT (autologous bone marrow transplant) costs up to $150,000 (and) patients must endure a horrendous treatment."* (86)

Then, almost everyone in the media — the doctors' and hospitals' groups, the scientists getting the big money for research, and the government health officials — went silent for 9 years. Nine years of a sophisticated breast cancer torture scheme which the authorities were "studying." While (of course) they simultaneously rejected and ignored brilliant breakthrough cures which actually cured breast cancer!

Finally, in March and April 1999, when the facts could no longer be hidden, the media reported what they, the insiders, "experts," and government "protectors of the public health" had known all along. Here's a sample of the March and April 1999 media truth-telling at long last:

> *"As many as 10,000 women in the United States suffer through the agonizing procedure every year. Doctors blast women with several times the normal dose of toxic chemotherapy."* Robert Bazell, NBC News Correspondent. (87)

> *"At issue is giving ultra-high doses of chemotherapy five to twenty times higher than normal, to treat advanced breast cancer. Those high doses destroy bone marrow and thus are fatal without a transplant of either bone marrow or marrow-restoring stem cells."* (88)

> *"Nearly 15 years ago, when some cancer experts began to promote the use of high-dose chemotherapy followed by bone marrow transplant, the results of four trials, the summaries of which were released April 15, proved (that) bone marrow transplant is not a miracle cure."* The Sacramento Bee (89)

> *"Current best treatment for breast cancer include surgery, chemotherapy, radiation and immunotherapy. Contrary to popular thought, transplants by themselves are not a treatment for breast cancer. They just enable higher doses of chemotherapy to be given than what a patient normally could withstand... They became common for breast cancer in the early 1990's. About 17,000 have been done to date."* The Milwaukee Journal

<u>Sentinel</u> (90)

"Preliminary results of five studies suggest the aggressive, high-dose procedure does not significantly improve survival. It remains a brutal regimen that brings a patient to the brink of death." <u>The Plain Dealer</u>, Cleveland, Ohio (91)

"Nine states have mandated coverage of the treatment, which costs from $50,000 to $150,000." <u>Boston Herald</u> (92)

"There is no proof that women undergoing the risky and painful procedure do better long-term than women given standard doses of chemotherapy and radiation." <u>The Detroit News</u> (93)

"Before the new studies came out, there was little evidence that the drug-and-transplant plan was effective. Even so, the process was in high demand among those with advanced breast cancer. 'There's a population of women who have been told that their only hope of a cure is a transplant, and I think we need to stop saying that,' said Dr. Lynn Hartmann of the Mayo Clinic." <u>New York Post</u> (94)

Bone marrow transplants were pushed for years by not just those reaping the $$$ as cancer drug specialists, cancer surgeons, cancer "researchers," drug companies promoting chemotherapy "cocktails," and government health officials, but also by women's breast cancer advocacy groups which raised large amounts of money year-after-year for their own breast cancer activities and agendas. This was done through marches and other kinds of media public relations events.

However, when the incredible results of Royal R. Rife's cancer cures were provided to these high profile women's breast cancer advocacy groups, what do you suppose happened? They ignored it!! It was too controversial! It might get them expelled from the political worlds they so enjoyed, the lobbying in the halls of Congress and corporate America, and on the television as they were interviewed. Tra-la-la.

What follows are what was provided to some of the biggest, most powerful names in the women's breast cancer movement. It got trashed so they could lobby for bone marrow transplants or fund "orthodox" researchers! Result: Thousands and thousands of women with breast cancer were tortured and died to benefit the cancer treatment monopolists and ruling class while fundamental, constitutional rights of individual women were denied.

Here's what was sent to critical "movers and shakers" — the story of Naval Commander Harrison's wife's miraculous cure of breast cancer in the 1930's San Diego world of Royal R. Rife. A Dr. Couche, who worked closely with Rife, used Rife's energy medicine approach to destroy the microbe responsible for Mrs. Harrison's breast cancer. Ben Cullen, another associate of Rife, recalled:

> *"Commander Harrison's wife had a breast carcinoma. The lower half of the breast was eaten away and she suffered intense agony all the time. But she didn't want to have it operated on because her husband had told her she would die of the metastasis and spreading it out in the bloodstream."*
>
> *"Well, he (Dr. Couche) healed her up perfectly and her breasts took on the normal shape. When she realized that she had two normal breasts again, it was marvelous."* (95)

But Rife's wondrous approach to healing breast cancer and other cancers was never permitted to develop and evolve. The head of the AMA was vehemently opposed to "energy medicine" or "electro medicine" or "wave form healing." It threatened the entire medical profession and its monopoly then, as it does now.

So the local San Diego Medical Officials were sent in to destroy Rife and those few maverick doctors who courageously worked with him and millions of women for decades to follow never had the opportunity to use the "wave form" medicine which worked so wondrously on Mrs. Harrison's breast cancer.

One foul deed, emanating from the ignorant, power-hungry, self-absorbed, ego-driven mind of the AMA head, protecting his doctors' union, devastated the lives of countless people far into the future.

Medical historian Patricia Spain Ward of the University of Illinois at Chicago stated the simple, frightening truth (the sunlight evaded by so many political leaders for so many decades):

> *"Morris Fishbein was instrumental in laying down the faulty machinery for evaluating cancer therapies which we have unhappily inherited."* (96)

FOOTNOTE: The <u>*Wall Street Journal*</u> of November 17, 1994, revealed the bone marrow transplant torture scheme against women on its front page! The money players, CEOs stock market sharks, business leaders, other mainstream media movers and shakers, banking moguls and legal beavers who run America, including the Clinton White House and "official Washington" with its pro-women political posturing, ALL were informed of what was being done to the women of America who had breast cancer. They all ducked, evading what had been exposed — full blown, front page — for the nation to know. They ALL ducked, letting those women in 1994-95 and women for the four and a half years that followed go down without a whimper of protest.

The <u>*Wall Street Journal*</u> article, citing scientific studies, declared the bone marrow transplant procedure — based on forty studies — was worthless and dangerously life threatening. The article quoted a leading doctor-researcher as stating bluntly, "*We found no evidence whatsoever that it provides any benefit.*" This was 1994, four and a half years before the breast cancer torture scheme exploded in newspapers across the country in March and April 1999

Why did this happen? Because the lead advocate was a cancer expert at the University of Colorado and Representative Patricia Schroeder of Colorado was head of the Congressional Caucus of Women's Issues. The cancer expert's data base was later exposed as junk. But, women's advocacy groups — delirious with their own power — decided to push High Dose Chemotherapy. What about the women who suffered and died because of this insanity? That was not the women's advocacy groups' problem! They were having a grand time exercising their political muscle until the results came in four and a half years later and the body count was a big unmentionable.

> *"Dr. Steven Narod, head of breast cancer research at Toronto's Women's College Hospital (stated), 'The optimism once presented by bone-marrow transplant seems to have dissipated.' 'Clinical trials of the procedure have not been promising,' Narod says. 'They're still dying of breast cancer.'"* Globe and Mail, Toronto newspaper, (September 27, 1999).

If you think the bone marrow transplant scam has ended, then you, the reader, are in denial and not paying attention to the clear message and warning of this book. It continues with various rationales because it makes a ton of money for the corrupt doctors and hospitals who promote it! Amen.

APPENDIX M: THE FAULTY MACHINERY

Patricia Spain Ward, the medical historian whose quotation closed Appendix L, was one of the most distinguished voices speaking out for truth in the 1980's and 1990's. While she is no longer with us, she deserves the appreciation of Americans now living and future generations still unborn who someday may benefit from her refusal to bend to the government health officials' lies or the medical rulers' phony pretensions. We'll miss her solid knowledge which served the American people's interest.

Another stellar voice with vast experience behind his words belongs to Patrick McGrady, Jr. He continues to reveal to mainstream Americans just how corrupt, stupid, and self-serving the cancer doctors, as a privileged group, really are. The common man and common woman of America unfortunately must pay the price for what the "ASCO tribe" is up to!

ASCO is the American Society of Clinical Oncology — the "chemo-nuts" fraternity of high paid sorcerers who keep pumping their poisons into trusting Americans' veins.

Patrick McGrady liked to nose around at ASCO conventions. What he discovered should be a wake-up call for an aroused democracy determined to end the "chemo-nuts'" tyranny. Here's McGrady's own words:

> *"I also attend the major scientific meetings, such as ASCO (American Society of Clinical Oncology). If you look at the American Society of Clinical Oncology abstracts from any meeting, and read about the drugs that are active, important, and getting good results, you see that the authors are talking about a few weeks, or perhaps a few months, at best. This may be meaningful to them because they never saw good results before, but the question of whether they get six weeks or eight*

ʦ or ten weeks of survival is not very meaningful to ..... patient." (97)

Now compare the "chemo-nuts" monopoly of cancer treatment with examples of what other medical doctors, other primary care health practitioners, and just plain common folks are sometimes achieving with a variety of Rife instruments. Here are two eye-openers among countless success stories occurring in many places:

> *"At the same time I started working on my wife's Abdominal Carcinoma, my brother-in-law received radiation on his brain tumors. He could not stand it any longer and asked me if he could sit in on the demonstration sessions with my wife. So we started, every day, from 20 to 70 minutes at the time. The tumors started melting out through his skull and scalp, as blisters. After two months, he went back for a second MRI and the four grape sized tumors they found very clearly on an MRI four months earlier, were gone! We have a hospital statement to that effect."*

> *"I have been interested in Royal Rife and his device for a couple of years and built two of them (and) have had excellent results. My father-in-law had lung cancer that has disappeared, a friend with throat cancer is in remission, an AIDS patient is showing no HIV in his blood, and on and on."*

Meanwhile, the desk murderers at the National Cancer Institute conspire to push their poison into healthy people! No longer satisfied with their "*faulty machinery*" inherited from the AMA and Morris Fishbein in treating cancer, they now have established a pathetic rationale for imposing their drug death system on <u>healthy people</u>! This is utter madness and evil, regardless of how clever and sophisticated it may be managed. The reader may not believe that it is occurring, but a short examination of the history of Tamoxifen (Appendix N) reveals the truth of what has been stated above.

Before proceeding into the dirty world and dirty medical politics of Tamoxifen however, let us briefly consider again the important issues which are known as "*desk murder*" and "*desk murderers.*" The source for the term is Nazi Germany and the bureaucrats who managed the trains to the concentration camps, carried out the vast administrative necessities, and so forth. Those original desk murderers have had their counterparts at America's medical agencies, the Food and Drug Administration and the National Cancer Institute, for decades.

Here's a quick introduction to desk murderers:

> *"'Desk criminals (Schreibtischtater). An important part of bureaucratic function is its sealing off of perpetrators from outside influences, so that intrabureaucratic concerns become the entire universe of discourse. What can result has been termed 'group think,' a process by which bureaucracies can make decisions that are disastrous for all concerned. Bureaucratic practice also contributes to the later cover-up of genocide by not only dampening everyone's response but also serving to hide individual perpetrators."* (98)

> *"'Desk murderers' could shuffle papers, set rations, draft telegrams, schedule trains, and dispatch personnel, resulting in the deaths of millions, without once seeing their victims or perceiving themselves as involved in the taking of human lives." (99)*

The "*faulty machinery*" (to use Patricia Spain Ward's apt phrase) created by Morris Fishbein's AMA and exposed by Patrick McGrady Jr.'s tales of ASCO shenanigans is certainly a form of "*desk murder*," given what is known and documented concerning the suppression of a variety of alternative cancer therapies which have cured cancer in the past and continue to do so.

Of course, the desk murderers dismiss such cures as "anecdotal." Without clinical trials, the "chemo-nuts" argue, no valid scientific progress can be established. This is a totally fraudulent argument with which they have brainwashed the American people, Congressional representatives and senators, and the media. As the careful, cogent medical scholar Robert J. Houston has made clear:

> *"The FDA requires a convincing mechanism to obtain approval for clinical trials, and I think this is a completely unnecessary requirement. If there are indications of benefit in humans or animals, that should bypass the whole issue of mechanism. The point is that the investigators do not have to know the mechanism in order to corroborate the effect that is occurring."*
>
> *"In cancer, case studies have a greater degree of validity than in other diseases... In cancer the rate of spontaneous remission is extremely low, so low that it is virtually zero. Therefore, if you have just a few cases, basically if you have two cases, you have something that is solid. So I consider what is being dismissed as anecdotal evidence to be, in cancer, actually an impressive area of evidence, because you can have much more detail in the case studies than you can in a clinical trial."* (100)

Supporting Robert J. Houston's dismissal of the clinical trial deceit is medical scholar Harris Coulter's devastating revelations regarding the fraud which demanding clinical trials for an alternative cancer therapy actually is. Here's a sample of Harris Coulter:

> *"If the controlled clinical trial were recognized for what it is — a mainstay of drug-industry and medical-industrial-*

complex monopoly — the antitrust impulse in American society would be directed against it today."

"The entire $550 billion American medical industry revolves, to some degree, around the controlled clinical trial. But because the theory is defective, the enormous superstructure erected upon it is equally shaky." (101)

So much for the AMA's and the "chemo-nuts" "*faulty machinery*" and their deceit that the clinical trial is the "*gold standard*" of medical progress. The case study method used to be the gold standard until the Ph.D. types at NCI and FDA switched to a phony clinical trial argument to serve their interests and not the American people's interest.

Tell the tens of thousands of American women who will die of breast cancer this year about the AMA and FDA-NCI policies while the women are getting worthless chemotherapy, radiation, and surgery because Royal R. Rife's energy medicine therapy which restored one woman's half-eaten away breast to full health was crushed by medical society greed and abuse of power.

Tell the American people how OTA (the Congressional Office of Technology Assessment under John Gibbons) conducted a phony three year evaluation of "*alternative cancer therapies*" and refused to look into Rife's miraculous discoveries, but did mention him in their report.

Tell the American people how the reliance on clinical trials results in children being tortured in ways which are specifically forbidden by international law!

Welcome to the experimental medical wards created by America's paper-pushing desk murderers. An example:

"Protocal 045 was an outrage."

"The study began in March 1988. Over the next two and a half years, three hundred and seventy two children, ranging in age from two months to twelve years, were enrolled at twenty-eight sites around the country.

> *Half the children who came had a totally worthless fluid injected into their arms — hours of discomfort in their brief and tormented lives, with no prospect for gain."*
>
> *"There were several justifications for the placebo. Some scientists believed placebos were necessary both to demonstrate the drug's efficacy and to remove investigator bias."*
>
> *"If Protocal 045 did not violate the requirement, set down in the Nuremberg Code more than forty years earlier, that medical experiments avoid all 'unnecessary physical and mental suffering and injury,' it certainly came close."* (102)

No matter, NCI officials insist on their gold standard. Dr. Peter Greenwald of NCI:

> *"The gold standard of evidence in cancer research are clinical trials."* (103)

This is utter nonsense and 100% wrong.

As long ago as 1986, Raymond Keith Brown, M.D. exposed and denounced the insane assumptions of the National Cancer Institute in a single and clear refusal to recognize the medical politics of what he contemptuously labeled "*scientism*." Scientism wasn't real science in Dr. Brown's mind. It was an aberration — a cruel, stupid, ludicrous perversion of good science and good doctoring.

Dr. Brown:

> *"Medical scientism ignores the empirical approaches of traditional medicine. It discounts clinical observation and enshrines statistical analysis, double blind studies and the prevailing consensus of opinion."*

The result is mass murder. The smart boys at NCI and FDA have destroyed countless families with their false dogmas and cute, insider politics, revenge tactics and absolute non-accountability to the American people. History will not be kind to them.

> *"Federal audit reports obtained by U.S. News show that the safety net designed to protect patients in research trials is riddled with holes at scores of institutions around the country."*
> *"Scripps Clinic (San Diego) was approving too many research experiments on children without following the special rules designed to protect them."*
> *"Medical care is based on the assumption that a doctor sees a patient as an individual and tailors one-on-one treatment. In medical research, a (clinical) trial serves the ends of science."* U.S. News & World Report, (May 24, 1999).

Clinical trials are sweet rot. Countless folks are being cured of cancer today through various Rife-inspired electromedical therapies while The NCI and The FDA ignore an incredible success story and the documented records, instead pouring millions of dollars into silly chemo clinical trials which produce zilch. A deep sickness, incompetence, and corruption pervade orthodox approaches and conventional cancer treatment and the mindsets and arrogance of oncologists and "chemo-nuts."

> *"Both individual patients and the medical establishment need clinical trials. They represent our only hope of overcoming the dreaded set of diseases we call cancer."* Robert Bazell, Chief Science Correspondent for NBC News. Quotation from Cancer Clinical Trials by Robert Finn (published 1999).

What can be said about Robert Bazell, based on the quotation above?

This can be said: He's totally brainwashed, totally unaware of other, valid scientific positions. He's also part of a continuing television network blackout of what's really going on. Stupendous healing techniques and discoveries exist which are blatantly, consciously ignored by those who determine through funding and medical politics what clinical trials by approved "old boy networks" actually take place.

Bazell is what passes for supposed expertise, informing the American people via a national television network which, coincidentally, lives off huge advertising revenue from drug companies. What a neat set-up, eh?

Chief Science Correspondent is a meaningless title given the worthless information put forth by him and the real danger it represents to unaware Americans who assume that the man is informed about the serious, life-and-death issue which cancer truly is.

A SOMEDAY LEGAL CONVERSATION (?)

"Mr. Bazell, did you actually write what was quoted?"

"Yes."

"Were you wrong?"

"Yes."

"Dead wrong?"

"Yes."

"While 10,000 Americans died per week, you put forth a fundamentally erroneous notion which encouraged cancer patients to enroll in clinical trials even though the evidence, factual evidence, showed most would not benefit from the drugs used by cancer 'volunteers' in such trials?"

"Yes."

"Did you ever report honestly and in-depth on working, alternative cancer therapies outside of the chemo-drug treatments which dominated clinical trials for decades at the time of your statement encouraging cancer patients to enroll in the clinical trials?"

"No, I did not."

What a sorry record — ten thousand lives per week!

The nonsense, lies, and tragedies perpetrated by the media science correspondents, uninformed Congress persons, and corrupt or incompetent or cowardly U.S. government "health officials" continues. History will not ignore their terrible transgressions against trusting, misled common people who make up the American mainstream. Two more media examples should demonstrate the issues clearly.

"*A Story of Courage: Reporter Who Chronicled Her Battle Against Cancer Dies At 38*" was the title of an article which appeared in USA Today on December 16, 1999:

> *"Cancer is such an epidemic, Cathy Hainer wrote in 1999. Cathy's story moved a nation, says Tom Curley, president and publisher of USA Today. Hundreds of letters (came) from USA Today readers who had been following her battle with cancer in the public diary she shared with them. Shortly after she began chemo, she began to lose her hair. She wanted the whole truth and she wanted it straight, not just for herself, but for all of the others who shared this disease."*

Dianne Feinstein is the United States Senator from California. Her commentary was published in numerous California newspapers in December, 1999. Title: "*'Tis The Season To Stamp Out Breast Cancer.*" An excerpt:

> *"Further research dollars are needed to conquer breast cancer. Each year, roughly 44,000 women will die from breast cancer. It's the leading killer of women between 35 and 55 — women in the prime of their lives. Also suggested are annual mammographys after 40."*

Senator Feinstein apparently has never heard of Californian Royal

R. Rife's cancer-curing therapy or the half-dozen (at least) other alternative cancer treatments which actually work but are ignored, verbally trashed, or outright suppressed by establishment medicine. Nor does she apparently have a clue concerning the quality science which shows conclusively that mammography is a political deceit and scientifically dangerous.

It's disgusting, isn't it? USA Today and a United States Senator, with enormous resources and research capabilities at their disposal, can't even locate what is easily — easily, easily, easily — found on the WEB if those running the media giants and the U.S. Senator's staff had the slightest inclination to dig an inch beneath the surface and an inch beyond what official science and official medicine was putting out (a phony, self-serving agenda).

APPENDIX N: DIRTY DOINGS — TAMOXIFEN

A good example of the mayhem and deceit consistently done by the "chemo-nuts" who rule the National Cancer Institute is provided by the history of Tamoxifen.

In the late 1980's and early 1990's, Tamoxifen (hereafter referred to as the "T-drug") began to be pushed as a miracle cure by the "chemo-nuts" at NCI. They convinced the National Institutes of Health Director Bernadine Healy that the "T-drug" could prevent breast cancer. Naive and self-absorbed Dr. Healy (whom Ross Perot in his deluded presidential campaign of 1992 wanted as his Vice-Presidential candidate) bought the "chemo-nuts'" "cooking of the books" and "rubber numbers" for their grandest clinical trial scheme of all time.

So, Bernadine Healy committed U.S. taxpayer funds of $68 million. Dr. Healy threw $68 million away to have the "T-drug" given to 16,000 healthy women, accompanied (naturally) by frequent mammography X-Ray testing of healthy women's breasts.

The problem was that the "T-drug" was known to cause endometrial (or uterine) cancer! No matter — that was ignored, not truly emphasized to the healthy women who were going to be the guinea pigs for the "chemo-nuts" at NCI. It was going to be a ten-year clinical trial!!! The "chemo-nuts" were ecstatic. The largest clinical trial in NCI's history was about to commence. There would be lots of money for research and committee meetings, paper and computer files to be maintained, conferences, papers to be published, and all the other baloney paraphernalia of a well-entrenched bureaucracy abusing its power and misleading the public.

The grand escapade — clinical trial of the century — began in the spring of 1992. Thousands of healthy American women began taking Tamoxifen. The drug company which owned it foresaw billions and billions of dollars coming its way in future years once the trial was completed and if FDA approval was subsequently gained. ($36 billion in yearly sales was one estimate.) Why such an estimated huge $$ bonanza? Because if all women 35 years and older who were worried about getting breast cancer someday in the future could be convinced today that the "T-drug" would prevent breast cancer, then the dollars and dollars and dollars paid for the worthless drug would flow and eventually flood into the drug company which owned it. Open the champagne bottles and ignore the massive deaths from uterine cancer which probably would result. But of course that required that the drug company's friends at NCI didn't get public virtue overnight. Not to worry, out came Peter Greenwald to push the "T-drug."

Remember Peter Greenwald — the clinical trial "gold standard" guy? He journeyed forth to assure the public about the "T-drug":

> *" 'No intervention is totally without risk, and tamoxifen does have some potential side effects,' admitted Peter Greenwald. He told the House subcommittee on human resources and intergovernmental relations that 'the likely benefits are a reduction in breast cancer."* (104)

A few years later, Dr. Norman Wolmark, the head of the clinical trial, despite statistics that by then provided gloomy results for the "chemo-nuts," stepped forth and urged women to begin taking the "T-drug" at age 35:

> *"Despite the statistics, Dr. Norman Wolmark, head of the study, advises women to start taking tamoxifen as soon as they discover they are at high risk for breast cancer. 'Don't wait,' he urges. Age 35 has been designated as the age to start worrying."* (105)

Wayne Martin, a highly informed cancer scholar and maverick who has bothered the "chemo-nuts" for years through a dedicated educating process carried on in various medical journals and health publications, warned the American public in the early 1990's of what was being done to women via the "T-drug."

> *"If every woman on Tamoxifen knew how bad the figures were, she would tell her doctor to go to hell. If you take Tamoxifen for more than two years, you increase your chances of getting endometrial cancer."* (106)

In 1994 the state of California declared the "T-drug" to be a known carcinogenic. This infuriated the drug company owner — Zeneca and ICI (British drug giant). They flew in "experts" to California's capital in Sacramento to lobby against the decision. (107)

But it was all smoke and mirrors, or sound and fury signifying nothing. Congress, the media, most doctors, most scientists, and the NCI and FDA "protectors of the public health" all kept their heads down and their mouths closed. The great clinical trial of the "T-drug" went merrily forward.

In October 1998, just 6 years into the trial, the FDA approved the "T-drug" for use by healthy women. It was approved even though the great clinical trial showed it didn't work! It didn't prevent breast cancer!

> *"There was no statistical difference in survival for the women taking Tamoxifen versus women taking placebo in the NCI study. An analysis of several large studies shows that Tamoxifen approximately doubles a woman's risk for uterine cancer when used for one to two years, and quadruples it at five years. The American Cancer Society and the media immediately hailed Tamoxifen as a breast cancer prevention drug."* (108)

Meanwhile, the drug company manufacturers of the "T-drug" began an aggressive public relations campaign to help American women become more aware of and informed about breast cancer! How altruistic and noble of them.

Zeneca and ICI, the drug company conglomerate which made the "T-drug," became the force behind National Breast Cancer Awareness Month (NBCAM), which is a yearly October ritual.

> *"Zeneca Group founded NBCAM. Tamoxifen accounted for $500 million of Zeneca's (annual) sales."* (109)

And all the while, Rife's cure for cancer as well as a number of other alternative cancer therapies which worked, were ignored or suppressed.

The "chemo-nuts" at NCI and FDA have committed crimes against humanity. Someday there will be a reckoning.

It is one of the arguments of this book that when it comes to the treatment of cancer, the doctors' organization (AMA), many health scientists, key government health officials, and certain private institutions and societies have been involved in murderous activities. The American people, for the most part, have not understood what has been happening, any more than they did in the 1930's as Hitler's Nazi Germany conducted its evil.

Yet, in time, America became aroused and went into Europe and liberated the Old World.

It is time to begin the educating process which eventually will lead to indicting those most responsible and their institutions for crimes against humanity. Why? So that future generations will not suffer as the people of America and the world have done, horribly, for the past fifty to sixty years under the drug medicine madness of the AMA/ PMA (Pharmaceutical Manufacturers Association) cartel and their sellout scientist/health official co-conspirators.

As one of the prosecutors at the Nuremberg Trial in 1946 made clear during his summation, describing why that special tribunal was established:

> *"By a declaration of criminality against these organizations, this Tribunal will put on notice the people of the whole world. Mankind will know that no crime will go unpunished because it is too big; that no criminal will avoid punishment because there are too many."* (110)

FOOTNOTE: Nationally syndicated columnist Ellen Goodman, July 1999:

> *"And what about drugs like tamoxifen, a powerful drug for women at high risk for breast cancer? It now appears in ads suggesting that all women are at risk. There is a difference between a cure for toe fungus and one for breast cancer."*

Poor Ms. Goodman doesn't even comprehend the basic issue that "*the powerful drug Tamoxifen*" failed in its tests. She is of course on target when she reprimands the Tamoxifen drug maker for its marketing scam directed at women consumers. But, regarding FDA's corruption and decades-long sellout of the American people by preventing therapies which cure cancer to be known and available — Ms. Goodman and all the mainstream media haven't a clue about that subject and haven't voiced even a peep when the documented information is easily obtained. Tra-la-la.

So the pharmaceutical crimes against humanity continue, the politicians smile and collect their payoffs in the form of campaign contributions, and the American political system — once the hope of the world — degenerates into incompetence, partisan phony issues, and rule by commercial powers and organized interests instead of "*government by the people.*"

Someday the Zeneca and ICI executives and their marketing boys, the American Cancer Society, and the mainstream media will answer for such dastardly deeds.

Justice and truth are not to be scorned.

What follows on the next page are history lessons worth noting carefully, especially by those who play fast-and-loose with the public in order to exploit or mislead people with cancer. It is clearly also for doctors, scientists, and government health officials who mistakenly believe they will never be held accountable. This includes the outside experts who sit on the FDA panels and vote overwhelmingly to permit toxic chemotherapys to be approved for cancer patients while the many alternative therapies, which actually cure cancer are disparaged and kept illegal, unapproved, and severely suppressed by state and federal drug enforcers of the existing monopoly.

William L. Shirer witnessed the rise of fascism in 1930's Germany as an American journalist. He later wrote one of the recognized great works on this human tragedy. The following is from a 1984 memoir:

> *"With horror I watched Hitler crush freedom and the human spirit in Germany (with) this Nazi barbarism."*
>
> *"I left Germany in December, 1940, fifteen months after Hitler plunged Europe into war. Britain stood alone. Not many believed that Britain would survive.*
>
> *"At the war's end in 1945, I went back to Germany. Adolph Hitler was dead. Nazi leaders were in prison in Nuremberg, waiting trial for crimes against humanity. Justice, at long last, had caught up with them."*

Allied warning a year and a half before the war ended:

> *"Let those who have hitherto not stained their hands with innocent blood beware lest they join the ranks of the guilty, for most assuredly the three Allied powers will pursue them to the uttermost ends of the earth and will deliver them to their accusers in order that justice*

may be done." William L. Shirer, 20th Century Journey:
The Nightmare Years 1930-1940, pp. xiv, xv, 617, 631, 633.

"'There are about 180,000 cases of breast cancer diagnosed annually and an estimated 75,000 of them need chemotherapy after surgery, according to Pharmacia & Upjohn' (drug company maker of a 'new,' FDA-approved and American Cancer Society supported 'breast cancer drug.') Los Angeles Times, (September 17, 1999).

"Why so much use of chemotherapy if it does so little good? Well for one thing drug companies provide huge economic incentives. In 1990, $3.53 billion was spent on chemotherapy. By 1994 that figure had more than doubled to $7.51 billion. This relentless increase in chemo use was accompanied by a relentless increase in cancer deaths." Dr. Frank P. Truitt, M.D., Ph.D., The Robert Cathey Research Source (WWW.navi.net/rsc)

"Cancer biostatistician Dr. Ulrich Abel, of Heidelberg, Germany, issued a monograph titled Chemotherapy of Advanced Epithelial Cancer. Epithelial cancers comprise the most common forms of adenocarcinoma: lung, breast, prostate, colon, etc. Abel concluded, after polling hundreds of cancer doctors, 'The personal view of many oncologists seems to be in striking contrast to communications intended for the public.' Abel cited studies that have shown 'that many oncologists would not take chemotherapy themselves if they had cancer.'" Ralph Moss, The Cancer Chronicles (http: //person.org/ chemolOl .HTML)

"Most cancer patients in this country die of chemotherapy. Chemotherapy does not eliminate breast, colon or lung cancers. The fact has been documented for over a decade. Yet doctors still use chemotherapy for these tumors. Women with breast cancer are likely to die faster with chemotherapy than without it." Dr. Alan Levin

"A (FDA) panel unanimously recommended expanding the approved use of leading cancer drug Taxol for patients with early-stage breast cancer. Taxol, sold by Bristol-Myers Squibb Co. is the world's most widely used cancer drug — 1998 sales of $1.2 billion. The panel voted 8 to 0 to recommend that the FDA approve Taxol. Breast cancer is the second most common cancer killer of women in the United States, following lung cancer." Reuters, <u>Los Angeles Times</u>, (September 18, 1999).

APPENDIX 0: HOW THE VILLAINOUS RACKET WORKS; CALIFORNIA CANCER LAW (SIMILAR ONES EXIST IN MOST STATES)

Now that the reader is familiar with the villainous and murderous tactics of the "chemo-nuts" who control the National Cancer Institute, and the horrifying results that cruelly, relentlessly destroy innocent families year after year throughout America, it is appropriate to expose how state laws and state government machinery work hand-in-hand with the medical villains in the federal government. California provides a focused example of how Gestapo-like processes work to keep real cancer cures from people who desperately need access to them. It is all very legal, of course. Legal, despite the overriding fact that California cancer law explicitly states the government's power derives from a clear, recognized duty to serve the public interest. However, that basis is evaded by legally enshrining the villains in an impregnable position where they control the process. "Yuck, yuck," chortle the "chemo-nuts" in their white power doctor and scientist jackets while they duck accountability to the American people and, specifically in this example, California citizens. It is very similar in most other U.S. states, and yet it is at the state level where the great possibility of blowing the villains into the dustbin of history truly exists.

In the health codes which legally govern California, the villains have truly established a mechanism which prevents any real alternative cancer therapy that works from being provided to a cancer patient. The law is insidiously clever in both its evil wording and intent. The key mechanism is known as the Cancer Advisory Board and is dominated by physicians, surgeons, and nonprofit cancer research institutes recognized by the National Cancer Institute.

So, there it is — simple, villainous, murderous, and enslaving. Classic treachery against ordinary people which permits the "chemo-nut" experts to continue their charade of protecting the public while actually, absolutely protecting instead their failed chemotherapy specialty. The hard statistics now overwhelmingly document the failure.

The law is so outrageous that it actually states that physicians must inform women with breast cancer of alternative treatments, but then goes on to restrict alternatives to "*surgical, radiological and chemotherapeutic*" treatments — what incredible villainy.

The rational basis (?) for this wonderful law and state mechanism filled with people and institutions approved by the National Cancer Institute is (of course) "*to protect the public.*" Here's the exact, clever wording:

> *"It is in the public interest that the public be afforded full and accurate knowledge and that to that end there be provided means for testing and investigating the value thereof of alleged cancer remedies, devices and informing the public of the facts found and protecting the public from misrepresentation in such matters."*

Given the documented history of the National Cancer Institute and the California Cancer Advisory Board, the above clearly means those institutions and the key individuals within them have failed to uphold the key basis for the entire law by squelching remedies and devices which actually do cure cancer. These people who make the decisions at the California Cancer Advisory Board and within the Department of Health have — through incompetence and/or corruption — committed horrendous crimes against humanity and atrocities beyond description by interfering (blatantly) with individual American's "*sphere of liberty*" in order to feather their own expert nests.

In defining how the law will be enforced by state police powers —

which draws well-meaning if thick-headed attorneys who haven't done their homework into being, tragically, accomplices to villainy and murder — the law requires that:

> *"The investigation or testing required to determine the value or lack thereof of any drug, medicine, compound or device in the diagnosis, treatment, or cure of cancer (must) utilize the facilities and findings of its own laboratories or other appropriate laboratories, clinics, hospitals, and nonprofit cancer research institutes recognized by the National Cancer Institute, within this State or the facilities and findings of the Federal Government, including the National Cancer Institute."*

The law then goes on to state explicitly that the Cancer Advisory Council shall recommend to the Department of Health which "*departments of universities, medical schools, clinics, hospitals, and nonprofit cancer research institutes recognized by the National Cancer Institute*" shall do the investigating by contract with the state. In other words, the "good old boy network" is protected against any serious threat by outsiders such as Royal R. Rife.

Such an insidious, evil game and treachery perpetrated on innocent, trusting citizens — giving powers to people who are unaccountable, ignored by the press, unknown to the public, left to do their thing by politicians, etc. — constitutes a wrong of monumental importance. The Cancer Advisory Board has forced deadly, useless chemotherapys on scared, desperate people with cancer year after year while simultaneously preventing cancer patients from experimenting or even investigating alternatives that actually do cure cancer permanently. Such evil is beyond any excuse.

The rest of the law is just cleaning up the bones. This includes:

> *"A violation is punishable by imprisonment in the county jail for a period not exceeding one year, or in*

> *the state prison, or by a fine not exceeding ten thousand dollars ($10,000), or by both such imprisonment and fine."*

And:

> *"County health officials, district attorneys and the Attorney General shall co-operate with the director (of the Department of Health) in the enforcement."*

It is not unreasonable to hope that someday, once the political winds change and the public recognizes what was done to them that — as with the Nuremberg Trials — past and present members of the California Cancer Advisory Council and the California Department of Health may have to explain why they ignored their obvious obligation to do what the law required: that the public be afforded "*full and accurate knowledge.*" Don't forget there are tons of public reports on the emerging alternative health therapies which the Cancer Advisory Council just conveniently never bothered to investigate, despite their absolute power. Accountability? Public interest? Citizen rights? There will be a day of reckoning.

A real accounting is long overdue, for the sake of justice, truth, future policy, and, out of respect for the countless victims who paid with their lives because of this infamy masquerading as experts just "*protecting the public,*" when in fact it was experts protecting their financial and career interests at the expense of millions of people.

Once it is all out in the open and widely known, the tall tales will commence from the doctors, scientists, and health officials, just as similar excuses filled the air after the Nazi concentration camps were no longer hidden.

War correspondent David Schoenbrun reminds us of a little history when the perpetrators of evil finally got exposed (from America Inside Out, p. 144):

> *"We never believed the Germans who told us that they did not know what was going on in the death*

camps. It was impossible not to know. The stench. the smoking furnaces, and the eyewitness testimony of those Germans who did business with the camp guards could leave no doubt, but they blinded themselves to the truth."

As have federal and state physicians, scientists, health officials, and ambitious Attorney Generals blinded themselves to the truth, resulting in torture, death, and a villainous treachery against innocent people with cancer.

Cardinal rule for government health officials:

> You don't play medical politics with people's lives — Period!

The following is a letter from a reader which aptly makes the point, grasping immediately the parallel between Nazi atrocities and decades of American medical genocide:

> *"From the first time I saw the kids outside of Sloan Kettering (cancer center in New York City) being rolled in for their cancer treatment, I knew that the use of chemo and radiation was nothing less than concentration camp madness. Imposing suffering of that barbaric intensity on anyone in the name of healing is undeniably evil. I guess what I want to say is, that telling the truth about the cancer conspiracy is one of my God jobs. I'd like to do what I can to help in this war against medical tyranny."*

APPENDIX P: THE DEPTHS OF DECEIT — MAMMOGRAPHY

The great deceit began in the early 1970s. It was concocted by insiders at the American Cancer Society and their friends at the National Cancer Institute. The number of women who were put at risk or who died as a result of this nefarious scheme is not known, but estimated to be huge. The Director of the NCI, at the time of this massive abuse of the public trust, later left government service and took a high paying position at ACS (sort of a payoff).

The American Cancer Society's self-serving program (financial scheme) continues to the present day (1999) and probably into the 21st century until enough women realize the stakes and force an end to the lie and the terrible dangers.

The American Cancer Society particularly wanted to push mammography because it could be tied in with the Society's own financial objectives (keep in mind the ACS slogan "a check and a checkup") and the radiologists, of course, loved the ACS program. There were few, if any, powerful voices — individual or institutional — which cried out, "No!" or "God No! Don't do this — NO, NO, NO!"

The collusive attack on healthy American women happened because the fix was in. Powerful politicians and the media were silent, silent as sleeping sentinels, while a determined, aggressive, self-serving gang of sophisticated operatives manipulated the nation's entire cancer program to suit its own interests. To hell with the millions of American women who would pay the price for the next thirty years or more, well into the 21st century.

In 1978, Irwin J. D. Bross, Director of Biostatistics at Roswell

Park Memorial Institute for Cancer Research commented about the cancer screening program:

> *"The women should have been given the information about the hazards of radiation at the same time they were given the sales talk for mammography. Doctors were gung-ho to use it on a large scale. They went right ahead and X-rayed not just a few women but a quarter of a million women. A jump to the exposure of a quarter of a million persons to something which could do more harm than good was criminal — and it was supported by money from the federal government and the American Cancer Society."* (P1)

The National Cancer Institute was warned in 1974 by professor Malcolm C.Pike at the University of Southern California School of Medicine that a number of specialists had concluded that "*giving a woman under age fifty a mammogram on a routine basis is close to unethical.*" (P2)

Repeat — the experts in the government were told not to do this to healthy women in the year 1974! The warning was ignored because Mary Lasker (whose husband was the dark advertising devil behind the Lucky Strike cigarette advertising campaigns) and her advertising/promotional/corporate power types at the American Cancer Society wanted mammography. Everyone else could go to hell. What Mary and her powerful political allies wanted in the cancer world, they got. Everyone else, including the public, was ignored.

By the early 1980's, NCI and ACS were at it again. They jointly put forth new guidelines promoting (again!) annual breast X-rays for women under age 50. They just simply refused to give up their lucrative racket. (One official candidly admitted the publicity brought in more research money for both institutions.) They refused to do what was not in their personal, empire-building interest no matter the cost in human lives.

> *"Doctors and their patients assumed that there was good evidence supporting those recommendations. But at the time, only one study showed positive benefit and the results were not significant."* (P3)

In 1985, the respected British medical journal The Lancet, one of the five leading medical journals in the world, published an article which ripped the NCI-ACS propaganda to shreds. It not only (again!) exposed the original onslaught by the high-level ACS-NCI conspirators in the early-middle 1970's against a quarter million unsuspecting American women, but reviled the continuing 1980's ACS-NCI propaganda.

> *"Over 280,000 women were recruited without being told that no benefit of mammography had been shown in a controlled trial for women below 50, and without being warned about the potential risk of induction of breast cancer by the test which was supposed to detect it."*
>
> *"In women below fifty mammography gives no benefit."* (P4)

But nothing happened. Mammography was known to cause cancer but the media and the health officials in the government stayed silent! The mammography policy pushed by the American Cancer Society to fill its bank account remained the U.S. government policy for ten more years until a massive Canadian study showed conclusively what was known twenty years before, but what was not in the interests of ACS and NCI to admit: X-raying the breasts of women younger than age fifty provided no benefit and probably endangered their lives.

In February 1992, Samuel Epstein, professor at the University of Illinois Medical Center in Chicago, a tireless opponent of the cancer establishment, along with sixty-four other distinguished cancer authorities opposing the status quo thinking, warned the public about the ACS-NCI shenanigans. The ACS and NCI (like long-married felons caught in a crime together) were outraged, terming Dr. Epstein's reference to the breast studies as "*unethical and invalid.*"

The next month, the Washington Post broke the story into the mainstream media (finally!). It published an article by Dr. Epstein which exposed what the ACS and their insider friends at NCI had done to countless women twenty years earlier and continued for twenty years until 1992. Dr. Epstein wrote:

> *"The high sensitivity of the breast, especially in young women, to radiation-induced cancer was known by 1970. Nevertheless, the establishment then screened some 300,000 women with X-ray dosages so high as to increase breast cancer risk by up to twenty percent in women aged forty to fifty who were mammogrammed annually. Women were given no warning whatever; how many subsequently developed breast cancer remains uninvestigated."*
>
> *"Additionally, the establishment ignores safe and effective alternatives to mammography, particularly transillumination with infrared scanning."*
>
> *"For most cancers, survival has not changed for decades. Contrary claims are based on rubber numbers."* (P5)

The crimes described were crimes. They were not errors of judgment. They were not differences of scientific opinion. They were conscious, chosen, politically expedient acts by a small group of people for the sake of their own power, prestige and financial gain, resulting in suffering and death for millions of women. They fit the classification of "*crimes against humanity.*"

In December of 1992, the New York Times published facts about the Mammography scam. The story included the following:

> *"Dr. I. Craig Henderson, director of the clinical cancer center at the University of California in San Francisco, said, 'We have to tell women the truth'"*
>
> *"Dr. Robert McLelland, a radiologist at the University of North Carolina School of Medicine, said, 'In our zeal to promote mammography, we as radiologists — and I'm one of them — haven't looked at the evidence.'"* (P6)

In July 1995, the prestigious British medical journal The Lancet blasted (again) the whole ACS-NCI mammography scam into global awareness:

> *"The benefit is marginal, the harm caused is substantial, and the costs incurred are enormous."* (P7)

But the spreading knowledge of what was going on made no difference to the bureaucrats protecting the public at the NCI and the FDA who had their empires to protect. Of course, the American Cancer Society furiously fought every attempt by those with any honor in the federal agencies who sought to restrict the number of mammography examinations for individual women or to extend the age at which a woman had her first one. Mammography was the American Cancer Society's "sacred cow" (cash cow) and they wanted legions of women to begin having annual exams as early as the ACS could brainwash them into doing so ("*a check and a checkup*").

By 1999, even celebrity poet Maya Angelou was shamefully and ignorantly promoting Mammography in public service ads on television, parroting the American Cancer Society's propaganda spiel.

Nothing had changed. Those protecting the public at NCI and FDA were doing the exact opposite. They were hiding, protecting their little empires, while American women were being needlessly exposed to dangerous, cancer-causing X-rays.

In September 1999, the full depth of the decades-long deceit was explicitly described in an article in the journal <u>Alternative Medicine</u>. It would reach relatively few mainstream American women who were being brainwashed by the "interests" through the mainstream media and pliable state and federal legislators ("*representatives of the people*") but, it did provide a torch glow in a dark night.

Here's the awful truth it stated baldly like a screaming American eagle to any American woman fortunate enough to read the hard facts:

> *"'Mammograms increase the risk for developing breast cancer and raise the risk of spreading or metastasizing an existing growth,' says Dr. Charles B. Simone, a former clinical associate in immunology and pharmacology at the National Cancer Institute."*
>
> *"The annual mammographic screening of 10,000 women aged fifty to seventy will extend the lives of, at best, two to six of them; and annual screening of 10,000 women in their 40's will extend the lives of only one or two women per year."* (P8)

So there's the lie and the depth of the Mammography Deceit spelled out: mammography will extend, at best, two women's lives for 10,000 women put at risk in order to benefit radiologists, the American Cancer Society, assorted bureaucrats, and other interested parties who profit off the vast, well-organized mammography deceit, when safe alternatives exist but are ignored!

That brings us back to the essential issues and fundamental principles which once guided the American nation into greatness. Which, of course, forces us to look again at the cancer empire's tyranny and threat to everything once held sacred in America.

The fine political thinker, Hannah Arendt, who studied the Nazi and Soviet tyrannies, and wrote brilliant works on the evil at the core of fascism and communism, scolds those of us who today surrender to the bureaucrats' conscious, unaccountable deceits and tyrannies.

Hannah Arendt's words:

> *"Bureaucracy — the rule by Nobody. Indeed, if we identify tyranny as the government that is not held to give account of itself, rule by Nobody is clearly the most tyrannical of all, since there is no one left who could even be asked to answer for what is being done."*
>
> *"Bureaucracy is the form of government in which everybody is deprived of political freedom, of the power to act. It enables him to get together with his peers, to act in concert, and to reach for goals and enterprises which would never enter his mind, let alone the desires of his heart, had he not been given this gift — to embark upon something new."*

It is time for women to try something new, such as the Thermal Image Processor (TIP) and to toss dangerous mammography, toss the American Cancer Society, and toss the ACS's lackeys at NCI into the dustbin of history. (P10)

P1. H.L.Newbold, Vitamin C Against Cancer, (1979).

P2. Daniel Greenberg, "*X-Ray Mammography — Background to a Decision,*" New England Journal of Medicine, (September 23, 1976).

P3. "*Mammograms Don't Help Younger Women,*" Spectrum News Magazine, (March/April 1993), p. 22. (Spectrum, 61 Dutile Road, Belmont, N.H. 03220—2525)

P4. Petr Skrabanek, "*False Premises and False Promises of Breast Cancer Screening*," The Lancet, (August 10, 1985).
P5. Samuel S. Epstein, "*The Cancer Establishment*," Washington Post, (March 10, 1992).
P6. Gina Kolata, "*New Data Revive the Debate Over Mammography Before Fifty*," New York Times, (December 16, 1992) (Health Section).
P7. C.J. Wright and C.B. Mueller, "*Screening Mammography and Public Health Policy*," The Lancet, (July 1995).
P8. "*How Mammography Causes Cancer*," Alternative Medicine, (September 1999), p. 32 (21 Main Street, Upper Level, Tiburon, CA 94920).
P9. Hannah Arendt, "*Reflections on Violence*," The New York Review of Books, (Feb 27, 1969).
P10. "*Thermal Image Processing: Breast Cancer Detection Years Earlier*," Alternative Medicine, (September 1999), pp. 29-35 (21 Main Street, Upper Level, Tiburon, CA 94920).

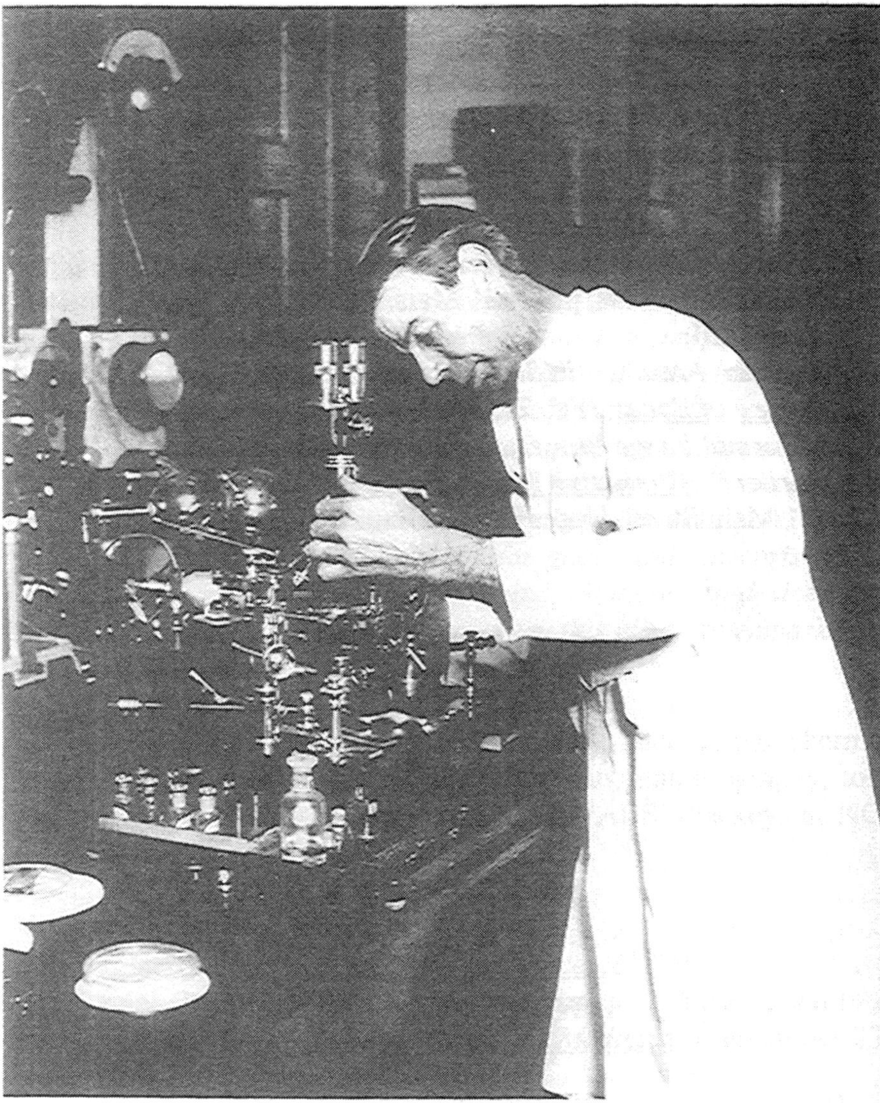

Royal Rife and his wonderful microscope

APPENDIX Q: BRILLIANT WITH LIGHT

There are people on the web putting forth various explanations relating to what Rife's "mechanism" for the cancer microbe might be, how it fits with current scientific knowledge, and so forth. There are also people proclaiming, from different cancer clinics and hospitals, that the Rife devices they have tested do not work as their proponents' claim.

The reader should recognize that these are classic diversionary tactics.

The mechanism of a cancer therapy, as Robert J. Houston's quote in ***Appendix M:*** **THE FAULTY MECHANISM** makes very clear, is not what matters. Does it work? That's the key question.

As for the fact that some Rife devices supposedly tested by cancer clinics or hospitals which are promoting their own, expensive, different cancer treatments haven't passed their tests, so what? Overwhelming evidence shows that some Rife devices are working and producing extraordinary results, as the two quotations in ***Appendix M:*** **THE FAULTY MECHANISM** clearly exemplify. The science behind the Rife therapy's results obviously needs to be understood in the light of modern knowledge. Also obvious is that standardized, state-of-the-art Rife instruments ought to be identified so that cancer patients won't be victimized by the trash black boxes. Emphasizing the negatives is an old trick of professionally educated elites. Even the growing Rife Revival movement has its share of educated idiots who miss what really matters.

It is time for democratic voices and individual patient rights to move to the priority positions. Let the nit-pickers stay in their pathetically narrow worlds of procedure and irrelevance! Let the rest of us get on with what counts — making alternative cancer clinics available to those people who want them now! That's what the public has wanted for a long time but the politicians and media evade the issue, serving the medical monopoly instead:

> *"Most Americans say clinics that treat cancer and other diseases unconventionally should be allowed to operate in the U.S. despite medical community opposition. Roper Poll."* (111)

> *"A recent Associated Press poll found that over half of the American public want alternative cancer clinics in the USA, whether the medical establishment approves or not."* (112)

Just consider the staggering possibilities of an open, mainstream linkage of Rife's technology, discoveries, lab techniques, and thinking with other, modern methods such as electro-acupuncture or other Energy Medicine approaches, plus the appropriate nutritional, supplemental and mind therapies, quickly determining what "mix" is working for a given patient.

If the reader can grasp the lost potential of the full Rife program in a medically respected, widely accepted, above-board, on-going, daily, creative healing process with the patient's full participation, then the crime of suppressing Rife not only can be viewed in its total iniquity, but the crime of the narrow, specialized, FDA-NCI-academia approach of today jumps into a much clearer focus, not only for Rife, but for other multi-therapy, non-drug approaches.

Rife truly represented a way for the patient to be actually part of his or her own healing. In each individual case, the direction of the healing would differ, as Rife's doctors demonstrated. There would be common procedures, such as painlessly destroying specific, disease-causing micro-organisms with non-toxic, wave-form Energy Medicine treatment. Keep in mind that Rife's research taught him how to take deadly disease micro-organisms and not only kill them, enabling a body to flush them out of the system before they did irreversible harm, but the research enabled him also to take some of the deadly disease micro-organisms and transform them into beneficial or harmless micro-organisms!

Rife:

> *"We have proven that it is the virus which enact upon the unbalanced cell metabolism of the body to produce any disease that may occur. We have, in many instances, produced all the symptoms of the disease chemically without the inoculation of any virus or bacteria in the tissues of experimental animals."*
>
> *"We have classified the entire category of pathogenic bacteria into ten individual groups. Any organism within its group can be readily changed to any other organism within the ten groups depending upon the media with which it is fed and grown. For example, with a pure culture of bacillus coli, by altering the media as little as two parts per million by volume, we can change that micro-organism in thirty-six hours to a bacillus typhosis (typhoid bacteria)."*
>
> *"Further controlled alterations of the media will end up with the virus of polio or tuberculosis or cancer as desired, and then, if you please, alter the media again and change the micro-organism back to a bacillus coli."* (113)

For four years, 1934 through 1938, clinics in San Diego and Los Angeles cured people of cancer and other diseases. The primary medical suppression occurred in 1938 and 1939. Rife continued his work into the early to mid 1940's, but with World War II (1939-1945), his primary sponsor dead, and official medicine barring doors previously open to him, the long descent into oblivion from the heights of national scientific prestige and wonder accomplishments produced Rife's tragic, unnecessary, politically-motivated eclipse.

In February, 1944, the Franklin Institute of Philadelphia, Pennsylvania, published an article describing Rife's Universal Microscope. The article was soon reprinted in the prestigious Smithsonian Institute's annual report for 1944. Here is one memorable paragraph:

> *"The predominating constituents of the organism are next ascertained after which the quartz prisms are adjusted or set. A monochromatic beam of light, corresponding exactly to the frequency of the organism is then sent up through the specimen enabling the observer to view the organism stained in its true chemical color and revealing its own individual structure in a field which is brilliant with light."* (114)

"*Brilliant with light.*" A phrase that says so much about Rife, his inventions, and what he still offers today if the scientific mediocrities, paper pushing government health officials and dark fixers or drug medicine corrupters in the AMA/PMA/medical academia world would get out of the way.

Dr. Robert Jacobs perhaps has stated clearly a truth obvious to lots of people involved in the Rife revival:

> *"The medicine of the future will be energy medicine. Probably 80 percent of medicine will be energy medicine, and 20 percent chemical medicine."*

Dr. Francisco Contreras, a Mexican born and educated physician who did five years residency in surgery and cancer therapies in Vienna, Austria and is now the administrator of the largest alternative medicine facility in northern Mexico, makes an equally eloquent, informed, and bulls-eye declaration:

> *"To me, the future of medicine is in light and electromagnetic fields. Once we find a way of manipulating and controlling electromagnetic fields, we will be able to cure just about any disease. Probably the guy who*

knew the most was Royal Raymond Rife." (115)

Near-instantaneous cures are where we are headed — regeneration on a scale now unimaginable.

"Out of the shadows of night
The world rolls into light;
It is daybreak everywhere."

Henry Wadsworth Longfellow
The Bells of San Blas

An affidavit filed by Royal R. Rife in the early 1960's included the following statement:

"Having spent every dime I earned in my research for the benefit of mankind, I have ended up as a pauper, but I achieved the impossible and would do it again."

Now, thousands are following in your footsteps, Dr. Rife, and doing it again because of the path you blazed — so brilliantly blazed with light!

APPENDIX R: LONG AGO WHEN THE MEDIA WAS HONEST

"PASADENA, November 20: Surrounded by the utmost secrecy during the fourteen years required to perfect it, what is described as the world's most powerful microscope, believed to be nine times as powerful as any other in existence, came to light this afternoon."

"The microscope, which medical men think will vastly widen the bacteriological field, was viewed for the first time by a layman in a small laboratory compartment at the Pasadena Hospital."

"As a Times reporter blundered into a small compartment, he was hustled outside so rapidly that he caught only a fleeting mental image of an unfamiliar instrument equipped with shining crystals."

"The new microscope is reliably reported to have a visual magnifying power of 17,000 diameters compared with 2,000 diameters said to be the limit of commercial instruments."

"By the use of quartz prisms, it is understood that Dr. Rife has broken up the light waves, making it possible to bring 'impossibly' small objects to view."

"Results achieved with the new instrument are scheduled to be presented at a meeting of Southern California medical men within a short time." Los Angeles Times, (November 20 or November 21, 1931).

"Scientific discoveries of the greatest magnitude, including a discussion of the world's most powerful microscope recently perfected after fourteen years' effort by Dr. Royal Raymond Rife of San Diego, were described Friday evening to members of the medical profession, bacteriologists and pathologists."

"Dr. Rife told of his development of the superpowerful microscope

and demonstrated it to the guests."

"The new microscope, scientists predict, will prove a development of the first magnitude. Dr. Johnson's guests expressed themselves as delighted with the visual demonstration and heartily accorded Dr. Rife a foremost place in the world's rank of scientists." Los Angeles Times, (November 22, 1931), page 1.

"Invention by a Southern California scientist of a microscope more powerful than any of its predecessors is one of the most important contributions to human knowledge. This microscope, devised by Dr. Royal Raymond Rife of San Diego, seems destined to revolutionize the whole science of bacteriology." Los Angeles Times, (November 27, 1931).

"The greatest advance in medical science since Pasteur discovered disease germs will probably result in elimination of vaccines and toxic inoculations as a necessary means of combating disease."

"The new polarized light, quartz microscope of Dr. Royal Rife of San Diego, (is) ten times more powerful than any microscope ever before built."

"The microscope, which had been perfected for years by Dr. Rife and used by him in his San Diego laboratory, was revealed publicly for the first time a week ago Monday. It had not been known even to the medical profession until a short time ago." Los Angeles Evening Express, (December 3, 1931).

"Using the new 'super-microscope' invented by Dr. Royal Raymond Rife of San Diego, Dr. Arthur Isaac Kendall of Northwestern University Medical school has seen, for the first time, the exceedingly minute moving bodies that apparently carry the life of bacteria."

"This visual demonstration of the hitherto invisible, living and moving particles of the filterable phase of a bacillus is hailed editorially by California and Western Medicine*."*

"The light used with Dr. Rife's microscope is polarized, that is, it

is passed through crystals that stop all rays except those vibrating in one particular plane. By means of a double reflecting prism built into the instrument, it is possible to turn this plane of vibration in any desired direction, controlling the illumination of the minute objects in the field very exactly." Science News Letter (Science Magazine) (December 12, 1931).

"Dr. Lewellys Barker of Johns Hopkins (Baltimore, Maryland), one of the nation's foremost authorities on internal medicine, is (a) visitor here."

"Dr. Barker had just come from a visit with Dr. Royal Rife, inventor of a new microscope which recently created a stir in scientific circles when it was found the instrument produces a magnification of 17,000 diameters, nearly ten times as powerful as others in use today."

"'He said scientists were claiming the microscope was violating all the laws of optics and I told him we would just have to let them get some new laws then,' Dr. Barker commented."

"'He seems to be a mechanical genius,' Dr. Barker said of Dr. Rife, whose workshop has been the loft over a garage at the A.S. Bridges home on Point Loma."

"Saturday evening he (Dr. Barker) will be guest at a dinner given by Miss Ellen Scripps, at which time the members of the county medical society will meet him."

"Dr. Sherrill, head of the Scripps Metabolic Clinic, is arranging Dr. Barker's program during the visit here."

"In 1899, he was Johns Hopkins medical commissioner to the Philippines."

"Dr. Barker, his books, papers and addresses, which are legion, command universal respect." San Diego Sun (January 7, 1932).

"It is the purpose of the report to record the more important observations made during three days, July 5, 6, and 7, 1932, spent in Dr. Kendall's laboratory at Northwestern University Medical School, Chicago. Discussion over these important, and in some

respects revolutionary, findings has become widespread."

"Examination under the Rife microscope of specimens containing objects visible with the ordinary microscope leaves no doubt of the accurate visualization of objects of particulate matter by direct observation at the extremely high magnification (calculated to be 8,000 diameters) obtained with this instrument." Proceedings of the Staff Meetings of the Mayo Clinic, (July 13, 1932).

"Dr. Edward C. Rosenow (Chief of the bacteriology division of the Mayo Clinic) confirmed certain findings of Dr. Arthur Isaac Kendall of Northwestern University Medical School, with the Rife microscope." Science News Letter (Science Magazine), (November 12, 1932).

"SAN DIEGO, California: Dr. Royal R. Rife has developed a combination microscope and micro-spectroscope capable of magnifying without diffusion to 31,000 times, which he hopes will extend the boundaries of knowledge still further."

"A little more than a year ago, the scientist completed in his laboratory here, the Rife microscope with a magnification of 20,000 diameters."

"With it he and Dr. Arthur L. Kendall, prominent Chicago bacteriologist, saw for the first time the filterable virus of typhoid fever, and, in another experiment conducted in Dr. E.C. Rosenow's laboratory at the Mayo Institute, the hitherto invisible bacilli of infantile paralysis."

"The new instrument, which Dr. Rife called the universal microscope, was constructed on the same principle as the first, making use of the variable, wedge-shaped prisms which were the unusual feature of the Rife microscope."

"The microscopes, perfected by Dr. Rife after eighteen years of experimentation, accomplished what even most physicists believed was impossible. They magnified 20,000 or 30,000 times, still preserving the image in its true form and allowing it to be seen with the appearance of depth. They also revealed to the eye unstained

cultures through the use of polarized light and monochromatic, variable beam, thus making it possible to study living organisms and those which resisted stain." Associated Press, (September 22, 1933).

"SAN DIEGO, California: A new, improved microscope, capable of magnifying without diffusion to 31,000 times, has been perfected here by Dr. Royal R. Rife, natural scientist."

The new instrument, which Dr. Rife calls the universal microscope, was constructed on the same lines as the first, making use of the variable, wedge-shaped prisms which were the unusual feature of the Rife microscope." The Christian Science Monitor, Boston, (Tuesday, April 10, 1934).

"Discovery that disease organisms, including one occurring in dread cancer, can be killed by bombarding them with radio waves tuned to a particular length for each kind of organism, was claimed yesterday by a San Diego scientist, Royal Raymond Rife, Pt. Loma."

"The waves are generated in a new kind of frequency device developed by Rife and one of his associates. They are turned upon the organisms through a special directional antenna."

"Rife thinks that the lethal frequencies for the various disease organisms are, as in the sound waves, coordinates of frequencies existing in the organisms themselves."

"Now, he reported, the mortal oscillatory rates for many, many organisms has been found and recorded and the ray can be tuned to a germ's recorded frequency and turned upon that organism with assurance that the organism will be killed."

"The discovery of the ray's powers traces back, Rife recounted, to a day eighteen years ago in his Pt. Loma laboratory. It was then his idea came to him. He has been tirelessly pursuing it to its conclusion down through all of those years."

"The studies now promise to revolutionize the entire theory and the whole treatment of human diseases." San Diego Evening Tribune, (May 6, 1938).

Following closely his announcement of the discovery of a radio wave germ killer, Royal R. Rife, San Diego scientist, yesterday disclosed scientific developments which have aided him in his intensive laboratory studies of the last four years."

Outstanding are four microscopes, most important of which is the universal model. All are constructed on new principles. A 'rush order' for one of the universal microscopes might be filled in two years, Rife's aides explained. A year or more would be required to make the blueprints alone. They would cost about a quarter of a million dollars each."

Associated with Rife is a corps of scientists and experts in the radio, physics and medical fields. The work to combat man's invisible enemies is coordinated to obtain the highest degree of perfection from each." San Diego Evening Tribune (or Los Angeles Times), (Spring 1938).

"Royal Raymond Rife, San Diego scientist, yesterday told San Diego club Hi Hatters of his experiments in bacteriology for McGill University (Montreal), Johns Hopkins (Baltimore), Mayo Clinic (Rochester, Minnesota), Heidelberg (Germany) University and London (England) University."

"Dr. Rife's listeners learned that he had done some highly involved research in tuberculosis, 'polio,' cancer and other cultures, and that he had invented and perfected the most powerful microscope in the world."

"After the luncheon he said his assistant, Henry Siner, is arriving in London today with a portable microscope to instruct the doctors and technicians of the London University in technique of operating the instrument. A larger type of the Rife microscope is now being made by him for those British interests."

"Next summer, Dr. Rife will go to London to deliver it." San Diego newspaper, (January 21, 1939).

"SCIENTIFIC MARVEL — Royal Raymond Rife with his newly

developed microscope — Royal R. Rife, of San Diego, California, whose home-built instruments have long been ranked among the finest in the world. One such virus, which the inventor declares he isolated with the aid of his microscope, has been found in cases of cancer. The intricately built microscope utilizes Rife's theory that organisms respond to certain wave-lengths, a theory he carried to finality by bombarding disease germs with radio waves which are 'tuned' to those of the minute man-killers. The virus he says occurs in cancer, Rife insists, disintegrated under such radio waves." Los Angeles Times, (June 25, 1940).

"Dr. Royal Raymond Rife, San Diego scientist, has been honored by leading American universities for his research and development of world-famous microscopes." San Diego Tribune-Sun, (June 13, 1946).

Mankind's long search for a cancer cure may be in sight as the end product of laboratory experiments conducted in San Diego fifteen years ago. These experiments and the discoveries they yielded are credited to Dr. Royal R. Rife." San Diego Union, (July 31, 1949)

APPENDIX S: THE AWFUL MAYHEM IN TODAY'S SAN DIEGO CANCER WORLD

The Scripps medical doctors of San Diego didn't like Rife in the 1930's. They saw him as a threat to their status and their kind of medicine and, since they were the medical powerhouses in that provincial little world, it wasn't long after Rife's historic announcements in the 1938 San Diego newspapers, regarding the Rife Ray's effect on cancer, that the San Diego Medical Association's muscle boys busted into the offices of any doctor using a Rife instrument and threatened the doctor with (A) loss of his medical license and (B) jail (confirmed by a witness) if the doctor didn't cease using Rife technology. Thus began the long suppression of Rife's wondrous healing therapy and scientific discoveries which lasted until the late 1980's when the Rife Revival began.

Unfortunately, the Scripps doctors are still the powerhouses in San Diego as the 1990's conclude and the 21st century begins. Thousands of cancer patients in San Diego have never heard Rife's name or been permitted to try his therapy. The Scripps doctors receive millions of dollars from the federal government and tons of money from private drug companies to test experimental chemotherapy on uninformed and misinformed cancer patients, not to mention the kids!

> *"Scripps Clinic (San Diego) was approving too many research experiments on children without following the special rules designed to protect them."* U.S. News & World Report, (May 24, 1999).

> *"The culture of clinical trials is plagued by conflicts of interest. Drug companies pay doctors handsomely —*

> *sometimes as much as $6,000 per patient — to test new drugs."* U.S. News & World Report, (October 11, 1999).

Now the Scripps powerhouse doctors are planning (plotting) a grand cancer center for San Diego which will act like a huge funnel sucking countless cancer patients into atrocious treatment and obvious conflict-of-interest clinical trials which will bring a ton of money to the Scripps Medical Mafia. Here's what the cancer patients receive: Organized mayhem.

> *"Cancer experts within the Scripps organization say they have put aside differences to form a major research and treatment center for the region."*
>
> *"'The main goal is to get everyone in the same system together on the same page in terms of cancer activities,' said (the) chairman of the new center's board of governors."*
>
> *"Another goal is to seek designation by the National Cancer Institute as a comprehensive cancer center — the only one in San Diego County."*
>
> *"Collectively, the Scripps hospitals have provided care for 18,000 patients with cancer in the past two years, which amounts to about one-third of all cancer patients in the county. The system also receives about $17 million in grants from the National Institutes of Health for basic cancer research."*
>
> *"Designation as an NCI comprehensive cancer center would not only bring in additional federal grant money but is a draw for clinical research projects on drugs, financed by private pharmaceutical companies."*
>
> *"Another benefit (would be) compounds developed by Scripps researchers could be tested in larger cohorts of patients."* San Diego Union-Tribune, (Thursday, October 7, 1999).

Meanwhile, in countless places throughout America and in other countries, people have been cured of cancer (documented!) with Rife-inspired instruments and therapies. Yet, the Scripps cancer doctors seek to build a centralized, monopolistic chemotherapy empire. Where are San Diego's political leaders of the 21st century? Laying low while their constituents with cancer are about to be chemo'd far into the future — Organized mayhem.

> *"'When you get involved with a cancer drug, you really don't know what's going to happen.' (senior vice president at a cancer drug company)"*
>
> *"'We give better protection to dogs than to people,' says C. Kristina Gunsalus, associate provost at the University of Illinois-Champaign-Urbana."* "*Dying for a Cure*," *U.S. News & World Report*, (October 11, 1999), pages 42, 35

Quality Rife instruments, which have cured people of cancer, can cost anywhere from $500 to $6000 to purchase, depending on the source. (Joining a group which uses them together can be free.) Junk "Rife" instruments put out by exploiters who put forth outrageous lies about the superiority of their useless electro-whiz crap units cost in the same range. (The Internet has a few of these despicable hustlers.)

Someday, standard, high quality "Rife inspired" Energy Medicine instruments will be common, both in millions of consumers' homes and in most healers' offices, be the healers medical doctors, chiropractors, naturopaths, nutritional counselors or some other category of front line, primary care workers. (Once our legislators — federal, state and local — wake up and honor democratic principles again.)

Unfortunately, the $500 to $6000 price range now can be (and often is) huge and beyond the personal financial capability of a desperate cancer patient, especially when it is an out-of-pocket expense and with no certainty that it can cure an individual cancer patient.

But, compared to the $20,000 to $200,000 per patient fee that despicable hospitals and stupid doctors scammed off women with breast cancer for over a decade in order to hit them with High Dose Chemotherapy and Bone Marrow Transplant therapies which didn't work and excruciating torture for a failed therapy that made tons of money and still is being pushed by the "chemo-nuts" today at unwary women with breast cancer — is there any comparison?

All the while, our so-called medical ethics experts and super medical research boys and girls remain tamely quiet in their quaint, protected ivory towers, not hearing or seeing the agony, terror and torture of what is being done to the average American citizen.

APPENDIX T: AND THEY CALL IT "SCIENCE"

"Pretend" scientists run our scientific institutions. Real, hard science — easy-to-confirm — resolving serious issues which confront our whole society are usually avoided and evaded by the professional "pretend" scientists. The examples are too plentiful even to list. Of course, the cure for cancer is near the top of the list of the "Big Taboos."

Science magazine is the most powerful, official voice of American science:

> *"Science, the new journal, began on February 9, 1883. Heading the publishing company was the president of Johns Hopkins (College and medical center in Baltimore, MD). The scope of the journal was broad. America's leading scientists were contributors. In 1900, Science became the official organ of the American Association for the Advancement of Science, and each member received the weekly. Executive editors under direction of a board have since been in charge."* Frank Luther Mott, A History of American Magazines, Vol. 4, pp. 397-308.

> *"'It's well know that Science magazine is very hard to get into,' says Floyd E. Bloom, the journal's editor-in-chief. Bloom is chairman of the neuropharmacology department at Scripps Research Institute, La Jolla, California."*
>
> *"The journal looks for 'things that are more than excellent science,' Bloom says. "We like things that are interdisciplinary, things that will have ramifications for*

> *a broad body of readers. We like things that change or challenge theory and dogma.' But even a minor advance stands a chance of getting published if it indicates 'there's another field here that we haven't seen before.'"*
>
> *"Science's Bloom is aided by about twenty staff editors. Their knowledge is supplemented by volunteer experts in new fields that develop, Bloom says. These experts read a batch of manuscripts each week. They answer the questions: 'If the findings in this paper were true, how important would that be? Would it change the field? Would it force us to revise theory?'"* Sophie L. Wilkinson, '*Behind the Scenes at Journals*, *Chemical & Engineering news*, (September 13, 1999), pp. 27, 30.

So the editor-in-chief of *Science*, who — coincidentally working at Scripps — sits in La Jolla, California, the place where Rife and some of the leading scientists of America cured terminal cancer in 1934-39, and his staff supposedly seek to publish "scientific" stuff that shakes the foundations of dogma.

Many, many people in San Diego and La Jolla know what native son Royal R. Rife accomplished there, but "official" science in America prefers the world not think about that! Does it all remind you, the reader, of a man named Galileo and how "official" science of his time just didn't want to consider that the earth just might revolve around the Sun?

Then there is that nasty little fact regarding the 10,000 Americans who will die of cancer this week, the 10,000 more who will die next week, and then 10,000 and 10,000 and 10,000, week after week on and on — trusting Americans who believe in honest scientist and honest cancer doctors who are legally obligated to provide the cancer patient with all alternative options regarding their cancer condition. Except, the scientists and doctors are not being honest.

Meanwhile, the official cancer experts at Scripps want to funnel all the cancer patients into one hot new program they are devising, centered around chemotherapy, plus, be paid a nice fee per patient for new experimental chemotherapy devised by the drug companies. Is there something wrong here?!?

> *"Since April (1999) when researchers first leaked word that high dose chemotherapy (HDC) appears no more likely to cure breast cancer than standard treatment, women who suffered through it — and the families of patients who died from it — have wondered: 'Why were at least 18,000 women subjected to this harrowing and expensive treatment to find out that it probably doesn't work?'"*
>
> *"Hospitals were only too happy to provide it, charging anywhere from $20,000 to $200,000 per patient."* *U.S. News & World Report*, (October 11, 1999).

Unbeknown (Purposely ignored??) to the "pretend scientists," many, many people with cancer have quietly been cured of cancer by various "Rife" instruments used by a growing grassroots movement of "Rifers" throughout the 1990's. But, the "pretend scientists" in academia and in their prestigious institutions such as Scripps, enjoying their prestige and fat salaries, would rather not look at the "*little, documented fact*."

> *"The greatest advance in medical science since Pasteur discovered disease germs."* *Los Angeles Times*, (December 3, 1931).

> *"The light used with Dr. Rife's microscope is polarized, that is, it is passed through crystals that stop all rays except those vibrating in one particular plane. By means of a double reflecting prism built into the instrument, it is possible to turn this plane of the minute objects in the field very exactly."* *Science News Letter*

(<u>Science</u> magazine), (December 12, 1931).

"In 1988, a medical researcher set out to determine if Rife therapy had any true value. We will call him 'Dr. X.' What he discovered was layer after layer of cover-up — publications with erroneous information (and) cards removed from the Library of Congress. Always the needed volume — sometimes only crucial pages — mysteriously missing from referenced sources." Rife source

Ah, isn't honest, open American science of the 20th century wonderful? Aren't you delighted that experts at <u>Science</u> magazine are working so hard in La Jolla and around the country to bring you, the reader, and the American public the latest, important scientific finding? There's this most wonderful bridge in Brooklyn that I have to sell you!

APPENDIX U: ASTONISHING WORLDS

From 1938 to 1963-64, it was known that cigarettes and tobacco were deadly, that they caused cancer and other diseases. Thousands of scientific reports documented the facts. The American press, in cahoots with advertising agencies, suppressed that truth. Millions of Americans subsequently died, horribly and unnecessarily.

The Surgeon General's report of 1964 was watered down into nothingness by tobacco congressmen and tobacco lobbyists. Only in the 1990's, after a courageous tobacco executive insider (Jeffrey Wigand) and a courageous Mississippi Attorney General (Michael Moore) challenged the foul, huge, criminal tobacco syndicate, did the syndicate begin rapidly collapsing.

The American Cancer Society was controlled for decades by the wife (Mary Lasker) and friends of the main advertising man for Lucky Strike cigarettes (Albert Lasker). The American Cancer Society was deeply involved in the cover-up of what tobacco interests were doing to the health and welfare of the American people. The result was murder and mayhem.

The Laskers were personal friends and card playing chums of Morris Fishbein, head of the AMA. So, the American Medical Association — the doctor's union — long kept its policies quiet regarding the health dangers of cigarettes and tobacco.

This astonishing little world of corruption and unspeakable wrong done to so many millions over so long a period has never been the subject of even a modern day newspaper expose.

Here's a factual overview of the historical, easily documented record. Read it and weep for the millions of victims — all because a few powerful people betrayed the public trust:

> *"It began in 1933. Under the direction of Dr. Ray-*

mond Pearl of the Department of Biology at Johns Hopkins University, a study of all deaths of patients from age thirty-five on, classified as smokers, light smokers, and heavy smokers, was begun to find, if possible, the influence of tobacco on human longevity."

"A summary of the study was available to the press in 1938 — the first life tables ever constructed showing that tobacco shortens the lives of every man and woman who uses it."

"Every (subsequent) honest report confirmed Dr. Pearl's 1938 study. It was now becoming a matter of life and death for many people."

"In carrying on a vast educational campaign for many years, the American Cancer Society and the National Cancer Institute of the U.S. Department of Health never gave the public a straightforward warning. At a time when the tobacco industry was spending millions on advertising and propaganda to maintain doubt and confusion, the organizations which should have led the campaign of warning remained almost neutral."

"President John F. Kennedy ordered the investigation of the tobacco industry. President Lyndon B. Johnson did not have the courage to take a stand. The tobacco lobby and its advertising agencies and their friends in newspapers, television, etc. emasculated the proposed law."

"Between 1938, when Dr. Raymond Pearl issued his study on tobacco, and 1964, when the Federal Trade Commission proposed truth in advertising, 7,000 scientific reports were published, all agreeing that tobacco was harmful and cigarettes killed and maimed people throughout the world."

"From 1938, the days of the first Johns Hopkins reports, to 1963, the day of the official U.S. report by the Surgeon General, ninety-nine per cent of the press

> *suppressed ninety-nine per cent of the news items dealing with false advertising of cigarettes."*
>
> *"Who can possibly say a word in defense of the American press which from 1938 on suppressed the tobacco-cancer news? The health and welfare of the American people are forgotten when advertising money is available."* George Seldes, Never Tire Of Protesting, pages 62, 70, 73, 75, 76, 143, 272.

Today the drug companies play a role similar to what the tobacco industry used to do — keeping the press silent through advertising agencies while keeping Congress contained through lobbyists and campaign contributions. Like the terrible, suppressed truth concerning cancer and tobacco, the new terrible, suppressed truth revolves around alternative cancer therapies.

How will the next generation of doctors react when they realize that they were mis-educated at enormous expense; that a huge amount of what they learned in medical school may be useless in a few years time and that other health practitioners, who receive training in fundamentally different methods and traditions, are much farther advanced in their actual, real healing skills? It is a safe prediction to say the young doctors will be (A) very unhappy, (B) possibly incompetent for the rest of their careers, (C) horribly in debt, and (D) perhaps the clients of attorneys for a long time to come in legal actions against the medical schools which defrauded them. Yes, they defrauded them.

The University of Southern California — Rife's patron institution until the great censorship and "memory loss" was imposed — may be one of the medical schools severely attacked by at least a few of its recent and future graduates.

> *"Said Clive Taylor, the USC School of Medicine's associate dean of academic affairs: 'Students may be thinking, 'Should I go to medical school, which costs $40,000 a year?'"*

"'Becoming a doctor is also an arduous pursuit, requiring four years of undergraduate study, four years of medical school and an additional three to ten years of residency training. Because of such lengthy training as well as the financial costs, medicine is not for those who want to get reach quick,' USC's Taylor said." "*Med Students Seek Cure For Debt*," Los Angeles Times, (November 27, 1999).

Especially if the medical students are taught "crap medicine" which no longer works and which a growing segment of the American people no longer want.

Meanwhile, many older doctors in the system are already in the process of switching trains and getting off the AMA-drug company clunker.

"More and more Western doctors are heading back to the classroom. Western medicine sometimes lacked a holistic approach, narrowing in on a specific illness or treatment rather than looking at the patient's overall health. The trend has been growing as patients demand alternatives to pill-popping." Dara Akiko Williams, "*Many Doctors Going Back To School*," Associated Press, (November 14, 1999).

Then, there is the "astonishing world" of Rife now surging into a 21st century renewal that — when it happens officially — will transform all of medicine forever. Let's take a quick journey into the past and see what was publicly reported about Rife before the AMA arm-twisted the press and media into censoring one of the greatest scientific and medical advances of all time.

"Rife is an expert in more lines than the average man has time to dabble in. He is an able bacteriologist, embryologist, electrical and scientific engineer, metal-

lurgist, chemist, (and) photo-micrographer."

"His greatest developments in the field of scientific apparatus, created during the past six or eight years, are:"

"The Rife Micromanipulator, whose flexibility outclasses any similar machine known to science. With this machine, an operation can be performed on a single blood corpuscle, as a surgeon removes an appendix, while the corpuscle is enlarged as much as 10,000 diameters."

"The Rife Super-Regenerative Ray which produces a destructive ray seventeen times as powerful as the X-ray for the treatment and control of malignant organisms."

"The Rife Refractometer, which has unparalleled flexibility for the measurement of bacteria, parasitic organisms or the prismatic angles of crystals."

"The Rife experiment on the weight of bacteria, which established the weight of a single average specimen at one-third of a billionth of a milligram. A milligram is the thousandth part of a gram, and it takes more than twenty-eight grams to weigh an ounce."

"He believes that the chemical baths themselves destroy the very germ that science is trying to pin under the microscope so, he is evolving a new method that will do away with chemicals. The possibilities of this process, once it is perfected, he believes, are boundless. Medical men may, in this one step, find an end to much of human suffering."

"This is Rife's great aim." San Diego Union, (November 3, 1929).

"A microscope is being used by a self-trained scientist in San Diego to wrest from numerous micro-organisms the secrets to some of the world's most baffling maladies."

> *"The scientist is Dr. Royal R. Rife who recently built the microscope and thereby attracted the attention of scientists all over the world."*
>
> *"Variable beams of monochromatic light are bent at an angle of incidence corresponding with the vibratory rate of the organism being examined. In this manner the minute granule, which is too small to absorb ordinary stain, is stained in its true chemical color."*
>
> *"Dr. Rife also has what laymen sometimes call a death-ray machine to destroy micro-organisms by impact at their own vibrations." "San Diego Scientist Builds Famous Microscope. Dr. Royal R. Rife Attracts Attention Of Colleagues World Over With Instrument"* San Diego Union, (April 16, 1934).

It was all there in the San Diego newspaper as early as April 16, 1934 — (1) the ability to destroy disease-causing microbes with a "vibratory" method, (2) the excitement of renowned scientists around the world, and (3) a microscope which shattered all the limitations of an erroneous physics. All of it was conveniently "forgotten" — pushed into a dark corner of history by medical, scientific, commercial and government agencies determined to maintain a status quo which was not in the public's best interest. Bad science and bad medicine thus resulted, dominating America for the next five or six decades!

Orthodox physicians, conventional scientists, supposedly accountable government health officials, and medical "ethics" experts of the late 1990's all continued to pretend that this incredible suppression of an historic scientific and medical breakthrough didn't happen — or was something they "knew nothing about" — or was dismissable as myth.

Yet, now the Internet and various other interactive, alternative medicine approaches blaze with Rife-related research and renewal of this great man's discoveries and the awakening and giant step into new levels of health — thanks to Rife and others inspired by him —

has just begun.

> *"Discovery that disease organisms, including one occurring in dread cancer, can be killed by bombarding them with radio waves tuned to a particular length for each kind of organism was claimed today by Royal Raymond Rife."*
>
> *"The waves are generated in a new kind of frequency device developed by Rife and one of his associates. They are turned upon the organisms through a special directional antenna devised by the two."*
>
> *"Eighteen years ago he began the studies whose reported results now promise to revolutionize the entire theory and the whole treatment of the human diseases."*
>
> *"Now, he reported, the mortal oscillatory rates for many, many organisms has been found and recorded and the ray can be tuned to a germ's recorded frequency and turned upon that organism with assurance that the organism will be killed."* San Diego Evening Tribune, (May 6, 1938).

> *"Three new and revolutionary conceptions of disease germs and their activities were disclosed today by Royal Raymond Rife, San Diego scientist, as a climax to years of exploration by him in the mysterious microscopic worlds of these little slayers of men."*
>
> *"The scientist worked for seven years straight and studied about 20,00 laboratory cultures."*
>
> *"Among the forms he reported isolated were those for cancer, typhoid, tuberculosis, infantile paralysis, streptococcus and staphylococcus infections and herpes."*
>
> *"Rife believes that the chemical constituents of the organism are so changed that it is brought within the visible spectrum, when examined in the special illumination of his microscopes."*

"'Moreover,' he commented, 'this special illumination reveals the filter-passing organism in characteristic individual colors.'"

"'So far,' he related, 'no two kinds or forms of organisms have been found to have the same colors.'" San Diego Evening Tribune, (May 11, 1938).

"In the world of health and disease, there are despotic influences that take incredible pains to hide facts that would explode their control over current theories and practices."

"It seems that the commercial drug and food interests have seized upon the mistakes of the pharmacologists, who long ago limited the useful and available drugs or remedies for disease, the weapons of the doctor, to poisons and poisons exclusively. The medical profession finds itself today treating starvation and deficiencies of mineral foods and vitamins with poisons instead of with the physiologically correct nutrient principle."

"Another great research man showed that one microorganism could be converted to another. With his power microscope that made live germs visible as clear as a cat in your lap, Rife showed that by subjecting the germ to a short wave frequency of the correct value, the germ immediately disintegrated."

"Local medical doctors who recognized the value of Rife's discoveries, and tried to apply them to their clinical work, soon found their relations with the local medical society canceled. No doctor was permitted to use his apparatus or methods on penalty of ostracism."

"There is still no general knowledge of Rife's epochmaking discoveries." Medical World, (July 1950).

The *Medical World* article was published in 1950, half a century before the millennium shift into the 21st century.

Perhaps the world is about to shift decisively, with Rife's long-lost science thundering its rebirth. Perhaps the new century will restore the memory of Rife's greatness and initiate the mainstream development of Rife's science as the terrible wrong done to him and the American people is corrected.

The correction of such wrongs has happened previously — throughout America's history, in fact. As the wonderful historian Paul Johnson reminds Americans of today:

> *"The story of America is essentially one of difficulties being overcome by intelligence and skill, by faith and strength of purpose, by courage and persistence. The Americans are, above all, a problem-solving people. They will not give up. They will attack again and again the ills of their society. The great American experiment is still the first, best hope for the human race."*

APPENDIX V: THE TYRANNY OF CHEMOTHERAPY

Chemotherapy didn't work. The so-called experts knew that simple truth for decades, but since chemotherapy was their bread-and-butter, they kept pumping it into millions of trusting Americans who had cancer. It was murder and no one in a position of power blew the whistle. One of the greatest historical tragedies in America's history occurred because a new kind of tyrant — a scientist-bureaucrat — had appeared on the scene and few recognized the deadly threat the new tyrants represented.

As early as the 1960's, the National Cancer Institute knew that high doses of chemotherapy were destroying the immune systems of cancer patients. The funding for the follow-up studies was canceled and the reports were lost or ignored. 116

High-dose chemotherapy remained an accepted, unproved dogma of cancer experts until irrefutable evidence in 1999 and 2000 made the strongest high-dose chemo supporters sink into their dark closets.

Thus, for more than twenty-five years, evidence had shown that officially sanctioned procedures had been killing people. Top scientists and physicians went along in order to protect their personal career interests. A form of institutionalized insanity had been at the core of these experts' opposition to non-toxic, alternative cancer therapies which had been kept illegal and ruthlessly squelched. The butchers of surgery, chemotherapy, and radiation had grown rich on the mutilated bodies of countless innocent victims while public health officials sold their souls.

Irwin D. Bross, Ph.D., formerly a top cancer researcher in Buffalo, New York, put it bluntly:

> *"There was little or no valid clinical data to support the*

dogmas that NCI and ACS promulgate in the mass media. In summary, the animal studies gave false conclusions that have caused unnecessary suffering for thousands of human cancer patients. Not only were the animal results wrong, they were used for purposes of scientific fraud and deceit. Moreover, this fraud has resulted in suffering and death for many thousands of humans." (116)

The respected scholar Harold S. Ladas, Ph.D. added this disturbing insight as to how the chemo experts got away with causing so much human carnage while deluding themselves "their chemo" would eventually produce results. Dr. Ladas wrote:

"In Oye and Shapiro's review of eighty studies in chemotherapy, it is difficult to escape the conclusion that such treatment merely appears to be effective because most of the studies (all but a few) did not employ an untreated control group. A five-year study by the Gastro-Intestinal Study Group (GISG) is a case in point. If no untreated control group had been used, the conclusion would have been that chemotherapy worked. However, GISG did use such an untreated group. Their conclusion was that none of the treatments worked and the data showed that chemotherapy also caused 5% rate of leukemia." (117)

Beginning in the late 1980's, "High Dose Chemotherapy" (HDC) masquerading under the public relations term "Bone Marrow Transplant" became a big scam directed against women with breast cancer. Ten years of this madness followed as thousands and thousands of American women were brainwashed into believing and risking their lives on a horrendous, expensive ($50,000 to $150,000 per woman) and useless chemotherapy dogma and therapy.

Finally, in April-May, 1999, ten years of this madness was exposed as nonsense. Newspapers throughout America finally told the public that High Dose Chemotherapy or Bone Marrow Transplant was worthless.

> *"A brutal regimen that brings a patient to the brink of death."* The Plain Dealer, Cleveland, Ohio, (April 16, 1999)

> *"There is no proof that women undergoing the risky and painful procedure do better."* The Detroit News, Michigan, (April 15, 1999).

This was a devastating setback for the High Dose Chemo tyrants running the NCI, but soon a foreign researcher provided hope for them. In May, 1999, his report suggested High Dose Chemotherapy might work after all! A reprieve was granted. HDC treatment of women with breast cancer began again.

Did anyone check out the new foreign super star researcher? Oh, that. Well, it took six or seven months for NCI researchers and officials to investigate. What did they find? The researcher was a fraud! He was a scientist hustler out to make a name for himself. In December, 1999, that little truth appeared on the back pages of newspapers as the foreign researcher admitted his fraud and resigned his academic position. Depression engulfed the NCI.

Then, in March, 2000, the prestigious *New England Journal of Medicine* published on its web site the rude truth that HDC was junk according to a new quality study which met that medical journal's impeccable standards. The final nail in the HDC coffin!

The Boston Globe on March 4, 2000, solemnly headlined, "*Last-hope Cancer Treatment 'Ineffective'*." The article reported:

> *"An aggressive and controversial form of treatment for advanced breast cancer has been shown to be ineffective, researchers said yesterday in a report that will probably end the practice of combining high-dose*

> *chemotherapy with bone-marrow transplantation."*
> *"Studies reported last year had come to a similar conclusion, but the verdict was clouded with uncertainty because one of the studies showed a benefit. That study recently was found to contain fraudulent data."*

The New England Journal Of Medicine, with offices at Harvard University across the river from Boston, Massachusetts, received $19 million or more a year in drug company (chemotherapy) advertising and had been a rabid opponent of all alternative healing therapies. It must have been galling for that snooty medical journal with its "impeccable" standards to be the High Dose Chemo funeral director!

> *"Why so much use of chemotherapy if it does so little good? Well, for one thing, drug companies provide huge economic incentives. In 1990, $3.53 billion was spent on chemotherapy. By 1994, that figure had more than doubled to $7.51 billion. This relentless increase in chemo use was accompanied by a relentless increase in cancer deaths."* (118)

Boston, one of America's leading (and stultifyingly orthodox) medical centers, was a big promoter of chemotherapy. It had a major scandal in December, 1994, when a health reporter for the Boston Globe newspaper died at the Dana-Farber Cancer Center because of a fatal drug overdose "through error." Investigations began. Outside experts were called in. The network of "prestigious" cancer centers around the country supposedly began examining their own procedures. A chain reaction ripped through the entire chemotherapy cancer world and spread throughout America.

Why? Because the media had put a temporary spotlight on the crummy, corrupt world of strutting peacocks known as cancer experts, who in their cozy, back-scratching world, kept the murder machine operating.

The experts squirmed a bit more when the Boston Globe reported the three hundred plus doctors and the three hundred fifty plus Ph.D.'s linked to the Dana-Farber Cancer Center, and the $167 million annual budget. All that supposed brain power, ethical specialists, "expertise" and money, year after year, and no break-throughs in curing cancer — Odd? — Smell something fishy?

The Boston Globe reported that Dr. Vincent T. DeVita was being brought in to head an "external panel" to investigate the accident.

But, the Boston Globe did not report — because it did not know and did not want to find out — that Dr. Vincent T. DeVita was not only the former director of the NCI, located just outside Washington, D.C., but also was the person who forced HDC down the American nation's throat as a national policy year after year. Nor was the Boston Globe about to report that High Dose Chemotherapy — Dr. DeVita's specialty — had been shown as far back as the 1960's, thirty years earlier, to destroy the human immune system and be especially worthless as a cure for cancer, especially breast cancer, which the Boston Globe's health reporter had!

Nevertheless, DeVita was brought in to assess the damage. It was a cover-up by the Chief Insider of the Chemo-Cancer World. The Boston Globe, mourning one of its own, couldn't even see the smoke and mirrors — or didn't want to.

The Chief Executive Officer of the Dana Farber Cancer Center lamented, but refused to give an inch on High Dose Chemo for breast cancer:

> *"It's just so discouraging. There's nothing we want to hold back. Do we and other places continue to do High Dose Chemotherapy trials for breast cancer? We think these trials should continue."* Boston Globe, (March 23, 1995).

Didn't he know (or dare admit) the sordid history of High Dose Chemotherapy? It was certainly obvious after five years of failure, even if it brought Dana Farber $50,000 to $150,000 per patient? Was he unaware of the studies from the 1960's which showed the National Cancer Institute maintained High Dose Chemotherapy for political purposes, even when the scientific evidence screamed it should be stopped? Besides, how could a person such as DeVita lead an objective investigation?

Boston, after all, was the site of the Boston Tea Party, Paul Revere's ride, "the shot heard round the world" at Lexington and Concord, and Bunker Hill — the beginning of the American Revolution. It was where Americans first proclaimed liberty over tyranny.

It took until 1999 — four years later — before High Dose Chemo as a cancer therapy was "officially" declared a loser. By March, 2000, the prestigious New England Journal Of Medicine, with its impeccable standards finally had to put the last nail in the HDC coffin. Coincidence of coincidence, in March, 2000, newspapers around the country carried the story that the 1995 scandal at the Dana Farber Cancer Center was at last "*all settled.*" The nurses who were found to be at fault had all resigned and the law suits were all quietly resolved — Those darn nurses!

However, a new, potentially dangerous story was building. A beloved ex-football player with deep community ties and involvement had been given one to three years to live because of the cancer ravaging his body. Thousands of friends and supporters had converged to encourage and help him. His team included the owner of the New England Patriots and the President of the John Hancock Life Insurance Company. John Hancock — the original John Hancock — was the Boston rebel who was the first to sign, in big, bold letters, his name to the Declaration of Independence in 1776.

So, where and how was this very special, beloved and admired person being treated? At the Dana Farber Cancer Center and with more chemotherapy! Already given a diagnosis of terminal cancer, he was put into the hands of chemo-cancer "experts." Just what his immune system didn't need!

> *"He was a football star at Northwestern (outside Chicago, Illinois) in the late '50's, and the first draft pick of the Boston Patriots. Know what the message is, the one (Ron) Burton's been talking about for almost forty years? Goodness. Basic goodness. Consideration. Kindness."* MetroWest Town Online, (February 2, 2000).

> *"Burton played six seasons with the Boston Patriots. He's inspired a network of doctors, business leaders, family members, neighbors, and inner-city youths who have concluded that it's too soon for Ron to say goodbye. They're providing the medicines and prayers he needs to beat cancer. Burton is one of the good guys. Almost too good to be true. That is why hundreds of people are praying for his recovery."* Boston Globe, (February 4, 2000).

Someday, perhaps, the people of Boston — where certainly one of the greatest political revolutions in the history of the world began (the American Revolution) — will recognize that another revolution against a different form of tyranny is long overdue. Maybe, just maybe, the spark might be struck (again) in Boston.

LAST WORD

The Townsend Letter For Doctors & Patients, a highly respected medical journal, carried the following on its April, 2000, issue cover: "*Children are being killed by chemotherapy treatment.*"

The article inside described how chemo-doctors lied to the parents of a two-year-old with a brain tumor. They told the parents that the Chemo treatment guaranteed survival. The problem would be raising the two-year-old "*as an ordinary child.*" Under no circumstances should the parents seek alternative cancer therapy, even one that had a good record with children's brain tumors!

But, the medical literature showed the chemo that the doctors proposed using on the two-year-old had consistently killed children! No matter — they poured it into the two-year-old anyway. As factual statistics had indicated would happen, the chemo caused massive tumors to appear. He died within days.

George Bush, the former President of the United States (1989-1993), when he was Vice-President in 1987, visited the site of the infamous Nazi concentration camp at Auschwitz. His response to that atrocity someday will be echoed by future Americans considering the outrages imposed by the chemo-cancer "experts" of our times. Vice-President George Bush' words:

> *"We went to Auschwitz today, on the 29th (September 29, 1987), and it was moving. How in God's name could anyone ever be so brutal? Could any people be so sick? God spare the world from this kind of brutality."* All The Best, George Bush (New York: Scribner, 1999), page 366.

Meanwhile, as the year 2000 brought a new century, in Minnesota and other states, superb alternative and complementary medicine legislation was being introduced as an antidote to the "old dog" monopoly medicine and its evils.

Even the AMA Journal's editor was whining about business ethics threatening "public health" issues. Of course she didn't dare acknowledge the AMA's decades of sinister "business" practices and crimes in her safe, little grumble:

> *"The ethics of business in a capitalist society cannot apply to the ethics of health care. Using business ethics without tempering them with the needs of society simply is not working."* (119)

Regardless of what the AMA officially said or did, the grassroots medical revolution continued to grow and surge — to the dismay of the "chemo-nuts."

Let us close with a special salute to Marvelous Minnesota! Praise goes to attorney Diane Miller who, with her Minnesota Natural Health Coalition allies, crafted one of the great legislative initiatives of American history. Someday it may take its place alongside the abolition of slavery in the 19th century and the achievement of the voting rights for women in the 2nd decade of the 20th century.

In February, 2000, Minnesota Governor Ventura signed the bill into law, effective July 1, 2000. The vote by the Minnesota legislators powerfully reflected the American people's long cherished, poll-proven desires, not the interests of the medical monopolists and health "experts." The Minnesota House vote was 110-23. The Minnesota Senate vote was 58-1. (120)

Now, other states, as well as the federal government, will have a model law to copy and Rife, Energy Medicine, and several other quality cancer therapies which work will openly, legally be available to millions now suffering from the dead-end, orthodox, super expensive, fraudulent medicine forced upon them by the medical tyrants.

> *"This is how tyrannies end: when people stop fearing the tyrant."* Jean-Louis Gassee, Los Angeles

Times, (June 8, 2000), page C7

All Americans should be grateful to Diane Miller and her revolutionary companions who sponsored this breakthrough law (Senators Morse, Hottinger, Samuelson, Berglin and Fishbach), the other Minnesota legislators who voted for it, and the pioneering Governor Ventura who signed it! The public interest has been served.

The dawn of a new day has come, but let us not forget the millions of victims from yesterday or neglect the need for both justice and vigilance in watching the old tyrants trying to keep their absolute, evil power in other states in the face of a surging, public demand for a "new medicine" that serves the public interest.

The Magna Carta of medical freedom for Americans has been written and signed into law! July 1, 2000 began a new world and, coincidentally, a couple of weeks earlier, the American Medical Association held its annual convention. One of the highest priorities for the delegates to discuss? "*Ailing finances*" and the fact that "*two-thirds of the nation's 800,000 plus medical doctors, residents and medical students*" now refuse to join the AMA! (Associated Press report.) Decades of murderous medical politics by the AMA perhaps were starting to have an effect on physicians who took their Hippocratic Oaths seriously and desired to practice the new medicine in the public interest.

NOTES

1. Morris Fishbein, *Fads and Quackery in Medicine*, pp. 299—300.
2. M. Layne, *The Koch Remedy for Cancer*.
3. David Wolper TV documentary interview of Senator Paul Douglas.
4. Ben Fitzgerald, Special Counsel to the Senate Committee on Interstate and Foreign Commerce, *Congressional Record Appendix*, (August 3, 1953). Fitzgerald was a highly trained attorney brought to the Senate for the investigation from the U.S. Justice Department.
5. Terence Monmaney, *Los Angeles Times*, (October 8, 1998), p. 1.
6. Chester A. Wilk, *Medicine, Monopolies, and Malice* (Garden City Park, N.Y.: Avery Publishing Group, 1996), p. 136.
7. Wilk, as per note 6, pages 181—182.
8. Wilk, as per note 6, pages 189 and 193.
9. Chester A. Wilk radio interview, October 6, 1997, KPSL 1010, Palm Springs, CA.
10. Ellen Ruppel Shell, "*The Hippocratic Wars*," *The New York Times Magazine*, (June 28, 1998).
11. Howard Wolinsky and Tom Brune, *The Serpent on the Staff: The Unhealthy Politics of the American Medical Association* (Los Angeles: Jeremy P. Tarcher/Putnam Book, 1994), p. xii.
12. James Flanigan, *Los Angeles Times*, (November 22, 1998), p. Cl.
13. Daniel S. Greenberg, "*Medical Research's Star System*," *Los Angeles Times*, (December 14, 1998).
14. CNN, Dec 17, 1998, 7:42-7:45 PM PST.
15. K.C. Cole and Robert Lee Hotz, "*Science, Hype and Profit: A Perilous Mix*," *Los Angeles Times*, (January 24, 1999), pp. 1, 23.
16. John Robbins, *Reclaiming Our Health* (Tiburon, CA: HJ Kramer, 1996), p. 268.
17. Charles Moertel, *New England Journal of Medicine*, 299, 1978, pp. 1049-52.
18. Shell, as per note 10.
19. Elizabeth Robinson, "*Essiac: Nature's Cure For Cancer, An Interview with Dr. Gary L. Glum*," *Wildfire*, Vol. 6, No. 1, page 48.
20. Wolinsky and Brune, as per note 10, pages xii and xiv.

21. Shari Roan and Terence Monmaney, "*Boom in Alternative Medicine Is Found,*" Los Angeles Times, (November 11, 1998).
22. Bruce Nussbaum, *Good Intentions* (Boston: Atlantic Monthly Press, 1990), p. 9.
23. Robbins, as per note 16, page 305.
24. Quoted in Scott E. Miners, "*Pioneering Physicians Hindered,*" Well Being Journal, (May/June 1996), (P.O. Box 1542, North Bend, WA 98045).
25. Evelleen Richards, "*The Politics of Therapeutic Evaluation,*" Social Studies of Science (SAGE, London, Newbury Park and New Delhi), Vol. 18 (1988), 653—701.
26. Arnold S. Relman, "*What Market Values Are Doing To Medicine,*" The Atlantic Monthly, (March 1992).
27. Lawrence W. White, M.D., "T*he Nazi Doctor and the Medical Community,*" Journal of Medical Humanities, Vol. 17, No. 2, (1996), p. 122.
28. David F. Horrobin, "*The Philosophical Basis of Peer Review and the Suppression of Innovation,*" JAMA, (March 9, 1990).
29. William Broad and Nicholas Wade, *Betrayers of the Truth: Fraud and Deceit in the Halls of Science*.
30. Dwight D. Eisenhower, Farewell Address, January 17, 1961, "*Liberty Is At Stake,*" Vital Speeches of the Day, Volume 27.
31. Ralph W. Moss, *The Cancer Chronicles Autumn 1998* (http://ralph-moss.com).
32. Wayne Jonas, "*Alternative Medicine and the Conventional Practitioners,*" *JAMA*, (March 4, 1998), v. 279, n9, p. 708.
33. "*Outside the Beltway,*" Orange County Register, (January 17, 1999).
34. Shari Roan, "*Two Pros Duke It Out Over Alternative Medicine,*" Los Angeles Times, (December 14, 1998).
35. Julian Whitaker's *Health & Healing: Tomorrow's Medicine Today*, (November 1998), Vol. 8, No. 11, pp. 3-4 (Phillips Publishing, 7811 Montrose Road, Potomac, MD 20854-3394; subscription telephone: 800-539-8219.) The *NEJM* editorial to which the quotation refers is: M. Angell & P. Kassirer, "*Alternative Medicine — the risks of untested and unregulated remedies,*" *New Engl J. Med.* (September 17, 1998); 339 (12): 839—841.
36. Dwight D. Eisenhower speech to Joint Session of Brazilian

Congress, Rio de Janiero, Brazil, Feb 24, 1960. Reprinted in Vital Speeches, Vol. 26.

37. My source for this Eisenhower quote is the Susan B. Anthony University Journal, (October 1975).
38. Relman Morin, Dwight Eisenhower: A Gauge of Greatness (1969), p. 138.
39. Alan C. Nixon, Ph.D., Past President, American Chemistry Society; quoted in Questioning Chemotherapy by Ralph Moss.
40. John Cairns, "*The Treatment of Diseases and the War Against Cancer*," Scientific American, (November 1985).
41. Sharon Bernstein, "*Drug Makers Face Evolving Markets*," Los Angeles Times, (January 31, 1999).
42. Office of Technology Assessment, Congress of the United States, "*Unconventional Cancer Treatments — Summary and Options — Part I*," Washington, D.C., 1990.
43. E. C. Rosenow, "*Observations on Filter Passing Forms of Streptococcus from Poliomyelitis*," Proceedings of the Staff Meetings of the Mayo Clinic, (13 July 1932).
44. E. C. Rosenow, "*Observations with the Rife Microscope of Filter-Passing Forms of Microorganisms*," Science, (August 26, 1932).
45. Royal R. Rife, History of the Development of a Successful Treatment for Cancer and Other Viruses, Bacteria and Fungi, (1953), pp. 1, 2. Rife's report is in the medical library at the National Institutes of Health, where it has been ignored by the high paid experts of the National Cancer Institute for decades!
46. Video interview of Robert Stafford, M.D. on October 3, 1998 in Dayton, Ohio describing his memories in the 1950s concerning the use of an original Rife instrument on cancer patients, research with rats, and a federal agency's attempt to take the instrument and study the research documents.
47. William Laurence, "*Crile Advances Life Ray Theory as Medical Basis*," New York Times, (October 9, 1933).
48. Malcolm Browne, "*Unlikely Results of Experiment Published in Scientific Journal*," The New York Times, (June 30, 1988).
49. Stephen Strauss, "*New Discovery May Explain Basis for Homeopathy*," The Globe and Mail, Toronto, (June 30, 1988).
50. Jackques Benveniste, "*What is Digital Biology?*" (http://WWW.digibio.com). Benveniste is a French scientist who proved

homeopathy's truth in experiments in the late 1980's which brought a hellish reaction from traditional scientists and questionable invasions of his laboratory from unqualified "debunkers." At the time of this writing (1999), he is the head of the Digital Biology Laboratory in Clamart, France. Mailing address: 34 avenue des Champs Elysees, 75008 Paris, France.

51. Popular Science, (1931).
52. Arthur W. Yale, "*Cancer,*" Pacific Coast Journal of Homeopathy, (July 1940).
53. Terence Monmaney, "*Nobel Prize for Medicine Goes to UC Scientist,*" Los Angeles Times, (October 7, 1997).
54. Royal R. Rife, paper dated June 1958.
55. Royal R. Rife, paper dated 1933.
56. Private communication, 1998.
57. Alan Blood, "*Rife Ray Cancer Treatment and Mycoplasmas in cancer and AIDS,*" (P.O. Box 128, Nathan 4111, Brisbane, Australia.)Available on web address: http:// WWW.ioa.comfrvdragonfly/pplo.HTML.
58. "*Royal Raymond Rife: His Incredible Cancer Cure and the Successful Campaign to Suppress His Work!*" www.healthresearchbooks.com/articles/rife.htm
59. Michael Coyle, *Advanced Microscopy for Nutritional Evaluation and Correction* (1997), pp. 13, 27, 241, 246, 252, 253. NuLife Sciences, 1321 Commerce St., Petaluma, CA 94954.
60. Majorie Maguire Shultz, "*From Informed Consent to Patient Choice: A New Protected Interest,*" The Yale Law Journal, Vol. 95, No. 2, (December 1985), pp. 293, 299.
61. Stephen A. Rosenberg, *The Transformed Cell*, p. 41.
62. Paul D. Harris, "*Energetic Medicine,*" Townsend Letter for Doctors, (August/September 1991), p. 633.
63. James Eden, Energetic Healing (Plenum Press, 1993), p. 7.
64. James T. Shotwell, *The Long Way to Freedom* (Indianapolis: Bobbs—Merrill, 1960), pp. 181, 371, 379, 381—2, 394, 395, 607.
65. David H. Hackworth, About Face, (1989), p. 340.
66. Ralph Moss, The Cancer Industry, (1989). Nuremberg quote from World Medical Association, Ethics and Regulations of Clinical Research, A. J. Levine: Urban & Schwarzenberg, (1981).
67. *Cruzan v. Director, Missouri Dept of Health*, Supreme Court deci-

sion, (June 25, 1990).
68. *Schloendorff v. Society of New York Hospital*, (1914).
69. *The Globe and Mail* (Toronto, Canada), (June 11, 1988), p. D4.
70. California law 1707.1. Cancer.
71. Lawrence Weschler, *Solidarity*.
72. Tom Clancy, *Clear and Present Danger*, p. 508.
73. William Bragg Ewald, Jr., *Eisenhower The President*, p. 138.
74. Alan L. Glaser, "*Alternative Healing and the Law*," *Medical Trial Technique Quarterly*, (Winter, 1994).
75. *Tune v. Walter Reed Hospital*, 602 Federal Supplement, (1985), p. 1455.
76. Majorie Shultz, *The Yale Law Journal*, Vol. 95.
77. Richard Horton, *The Lancet*, (March 6, 1933).
78. Bernard Cohen, *Revolution in Science*.
79. James DeMeo, "*More FDA 'Ban and Burn' Actions*," (26 Sep 1998). (obrl-news@lists.village.virginia.edu) Postal mailing address: Orgone Biophysical Research Laboratory, Inc., Greensprings Center, P.O. Box 1148, Ashland, OR 97520.
80. Jacob Liberman, *Light: Medicine of the Future*.
81. Loren Biser, *The Layman's Course on Killing Cancer*.
82. John W. Cartmell, "*Cancer: A Paradigm and Protocol*," published without protocol in *Frontier Perspectives* (Spring/Summer 1997); reprinted in *Townsend Letter for Doctors and Patients*, (Feb/Mar 1998) and again in *SunCoast ECO Report*, (Aug/Sep 1998), (P.O. Box 35500, SunCoast, FL 34278, $24 for 10 issues; a not for profit tax-exempt corporation. Contributions are tax deductible.) A protocol worthy of serious scientific testing?!
83. The Hippocratic Oath
84. Chief Justice of the Supreme Court William Rehnquist, *Cruzan v. Director, Missouri Dept of Health*, (June 25, 1990).
85. Associate Justice William Brennan, *Cruzan v. Director, Missouri Dept of Health*, (June 25, 1990).
86. Melinda Beck, "*The Politics of Breast Cancer*," *Newsweek* (December 10, 1990).
87. Robert Bazell, "*Bone Marrow Transplants May Not Work For Breast Cancer*," MSNBC web site, (March 9, 1999).
88. "*Bone Marrow Swap in Breast Cancer Still in Question*," *The London Free Press*, (April 19, 1999), from Associated Press and

The Toronto Sun.

89. David M. Eddy and Craig Henderson, "*Bone Marrow Transplants: No Breast Cancer Miracle Cure*," The Sacramento Bee, California, (April 20, 1999).
90. Marilyn Marchione, "*What's Next for treatment?*", The Milwaukee Journal Sentinel, Wisconsin, (April 18, 1999).
91. Harlan Spector and Diane Solov, "*Breast Cancer Patients Still Face Choice, Transplant Offers No Clear Benefit, Five Studies Show*," The Plain Dealer, Cleveland, Ohio, (April 16, 1999).
92. Michael Lasalandra, "*Breast Cancer Studies Extend Treatment Debate*," Boston Herald, Massachusetts, (April 16, 1999).
93. Lauran Neergaard, Associated Press, "*Costly New Breast Cancer Treatment May Not Work*," The Detroit News, Michigan, (April 15, 1999).
94. "*Breast Cancer Quakery*," New York Post, (April 20, 1999).
95. Ben Cullen, transcript of interview, October 15, 1959.
96. Ken Ausubel, "*The Silent Treatments*," New Age Journal, (September/October, 1989), p. 117.
97. David J. Hess, *Evaluating Alternative Cancer Therapies: A Guide to the Science and Politics of an Emerging Medical Field*, (Piscataway, N.J.: Rutgers University Press, 1999), pp. 28, 30—31.
98. Robert Jay Lifton, *The Nazi Doctors: Medical Killing and the Psychology of Killing* (Basic Books), pp. 60, 496, 497.
99. Christopher R. Browning, from *Critical Issues of the Holocaust*, edited by Alex Grabman and Daniel Landes (1983).
100. Hess, per note 97, pp. 132, 135.
101. Harris L. Coulter, *The Controlled Clinical Trial* (Washington, D.C.: Center for Empirical Medicine, 1991).
102. Peter Arno and Karyn Feiden, *Against the Odds* (Harperdollins, 1992), p. 204.
103. Reported by Associated Press and published in the *Los Angeles Times*, (March 15,1993).
104. Ralph W. Moss, *The Cancer Chronicles #14*, (February, 1993).
105. "*Tamoxifen: Cancer Causing Drug Approved for Healthy Women*," *Life Extension*, (May, 1999), p. 16.
106. Wayne Martin, from an interview in *The Layman's Course on Killing Cancer* by Loren Biser, Section 33, pp. 4-5.
107. Ralph W. Moss, *The Cancer Chronicles #30*, (December 1995).

108. "*Tamoxifen.. .*", as per note 105, pp. 15, 16, 19.
109. "T*hings that Make You Go Hmm*," *Well Being Journal*, (January/ February 1999), (P.O. Box 1542, North Bend, WA 98045-1542), pp. 19, 25.
110. Telford Taylor, *The Anatomy of the Nuremberg Trials*,(New York: Knopf, 1992), p. 527.
111. "*Cancer Clinics*," *The Houston Post*, (May 9, 1990).
112. Harold Ladas, "*The War On Cancer*," *Holistic Medicine*, Vol. 3 (London, 1988).
113. Royal Rife, *History of the Development of a Successful Treatment for Cancer and Other Viruses, Bacteria and Fungi* (1953), pp. 3, 4, 12.
114. R. E. Seidel and M. Elizabeth Winter, "*The New Microscopes*," *Journal of the Franklin Institute*, Philadelphia, PA, (February 1944), pp. 117-118. Reprinted in *The Smithsonian Institute's Annual Report*, (1944).
115. Hess, as per note 97, pp. 94, 101.
116. Irwin Bross, "*Mathematical Models vs. Animal Models*," *Perspective on Animal Research*, Vol. 1, (1988). Medical Research Modernization Committee, P. O. Box 6036, Grand Central Station, New York, NY. Dr. Bross also authored *Crimes of Official Science*, Biomedical Metatechnology Press, Buffalo, NY, (1988).
117. Harold S. Ladas, Ph.D., "*The war on Cancer: Victory or Deadlock?*", *Holistic Medicine*, Vol. 3, (1988).
118. Frank P. Truitt, M.D., Ph.D., *The Robert Cathey Research Source*, Web address: www.navi.net/rsc.
119. *Los Angeles Times*, (May 5, 2000), page A28.
120. *The Complementary and Alternative Health Freedom of Access Act.* The test from hereon is to keep the fundamental structure and purpose of the Minnesota law as the model for both other states and, eventually, a national law covering the entire medical treatment rights for all Americans. Have no illusions about the AMA, drug companies, government health cronyism, scientific "elites" and others using lobbyists and $$$ to alter the original rights and turn them into paper words meaning nothing. Vigilance!